Atlas of Renal Pathology

Current Histopathology

Consultant Editor
Professor G. Austin Gresham, TD, ScD, MD, FRC Path.
Professor of Morbid Anatomy and Histology, University of Cambridge

Volume Two

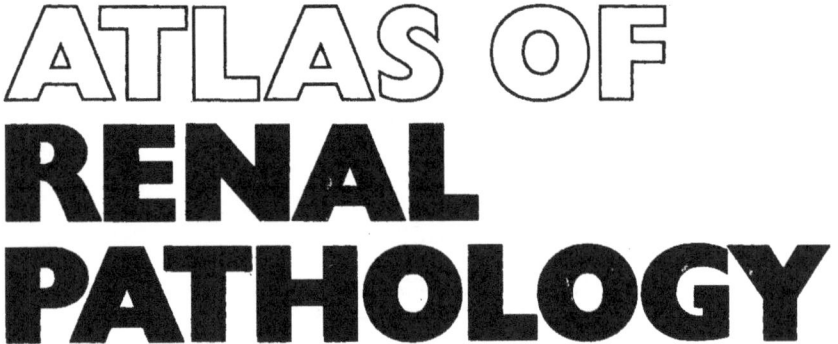

RENAL PATHOLOGY

BY R. A. RISDON

Reader in Morbid Anatomy and Honorary Consultant Pathologist
The London Hospital Medical College

AND D. R. TURNER

Reader in Pathology and Honorary Consultant Pathologist
Guy's Hospital Medical School, London

Springer-Science+Business Media, B.V.

Copyright © 1980 Springer Science+Business Media Dordrecht
Originally published by MTP Press Limited in 1980
Softcover reprint of the hardcover 1st edition 1980

British Library Cataloguing in Publication Data

Risdon, R A
   Atlas of renal pathology.–(Current
   histopathology series; vol. 2).
   1. Kidneys–Diseases
   I. Title   II. Turner, D R   III. Series
   616.6'1'07   RC904

   ISBN 978-94-009-8691-6   ISBN 978-94-009-8689-3 (eBook)
   DOI 10.1007/978-94-009-8689-3

Contents

Current Histopathology Series

Consultant Editor's Note

At the present time books on morbid anatomy and histology can be divided into two broad groups: extensive textbooks often written primarily for students and monographs on research topics.

This takes no account of the fact that the vast majority of pathologists are involved in an essentially practical field of general Diagnostic Pathology, providing an important service to their clinical colleagues. Many of these pathologists are expected to cover a broad range of disciplines and even those who remain solely within the field of histopathology usually have single and sole responsibility within the hospital for all this work. They may often have no chance for direct discussion on problem cases with colleagues in the same department. In the field of histopathology, no less than in other medical fields, there have been extensive and recent advances, not only in new histochemical techniques but also in the type of specimen provided by new surgical procedures.

There is a great need for the provision of appropriate information for this group. This need has been defined in the following terms.

1. It should be aimed at the general clinical pathologist or histopathologist with existing practical training, but should also have value for the trainee pathologist.
2. It should concentrate on the practical aspects of histopathology taking account of the new techniques which should be within the compass of the worker in a unit with reasonable facilities.
3. New types of material e.g. those derived from endoscopic biopsy should be covered fully.
4. There should be an adequate number of illustrations on each subject to demonstrate the variation in appearance that is encountered.
5. Colour illustrations should be used wherever they aid recognition.

The present concept stemmed from this definition but it was immediately realized that these aims could only be achieved within the compass of a series, of which this volume is one. Since histopathology is, by its very nature, systematized, the individual volumes deal with one system or where this appears more appropriate with a single organ.

Several volumes of this series of current histopathology are now being prepared. This is the second volume of the series; the first volume appeared in January 1980 and has been accepted as a valuable bench manual for the histopathologist. The design and content of this second volume on renal pathology has the same aims in view and will, without doubt, achieve them. The authors have selected topics which often provide problems for the diagnostic histopathologist. The concise text coupled with comprehensive illustrations is a model for the series.

G. Austin Gresham
Cambridge

Introduction

This book is intended as a practical bench manual for the hospital pathologist who wishes to have access to a simple informative account of renal pathology, particularly for the interpretation of percutaneous needle biopsy specimens. In addition we trust it will be valuable to physicians working in the field of renal disease, for whom the interpretation of renal biopsy material is directly relevant to patient management.

Whilst a comprehensive coverage more appropriate to a larger text has not been attempted, the text has been planned to give an adequate account of the more important non-neoplastic disease processes and their pathological appearances in the kidney. Points of difficulty in interpretation and differential diagnosis are covered both in the text and in the illustrations. Special staining techniques, immunofluorescence, and immunoperoxidase methods, electron microscopy and the use of plastic-embedded sections for light microscopy are often useful and occasionally vital in identifying the morphological abnormalities in renal diseases, and where appropriate these have been illustrated.

Although the main emphasis is on the pathology, the relevant clinical aspects of the conditions covered are included in recognition of the fact that renal disease is an area in which correlation of the clinical and histopathological findings is particularly important in reaching an informed diagnosis.

Acknowledgements

We would like to thank the technical staff of the Histopathology Laboratories of The London Hospital Medical College, The Hospital for Sick Children, Great Ormond Street, and Guy's Hospital Medical School for the preparation of the sections from which the majority of the illustrations have been made, the staffs of the Medical Illustration Departments of these institutions for their help and advice, and Rose Heron who typed the manuscript.

The functional units of the kidney are the nephrons of which about a million are present in each organ. Each nephron consists of a tubule (about 50 mm long and between 20 and 50 μm in diameter) with a lobulated tuft of specialized capillaries at the expanded blind proximal end which forms the glomerulus. Blood flow to the kidneys is large in relation to their size and about one-fifth of the plasma volume passing through the kidneys is filtered through the glomerular capillary walls to produce a nearly protein-free glomerular filtrate. This is modified by selective reabsorption and secretion during its passage through the tubules to form urine. The various mechanisms controlling this process help to maintain the normal volume and constitution of the extracellular fluid.

Glomerulus

The glomerular tuft capillaries are supplied with blood by an *afferent arteriole* and drained by an *efferent arteriole*. Within the tuft the capillaries are grouped in *lobules*; in histological sections, the capillaries are often cut obliquely so that their cross-sectional profiles are oval, irregularly curved or sometimes branched. The glomerular tuft lies in a spherical space (the *urinary space*) bounded by *Bowman's capsule*. This consists of a basement membrane lined by flattened epithelial cells (Figures 1.1 and 1.2).

The capillaries of the glomerular tuft have a continuous *basement membrane* (GBM) common to all the loops. This consists of three layers, a central electron-dense layer (the *lamina densa*) between two less electron-dense layers (the *lamina rara interna* and *externa*) (Figure 1.3). The prominence of the three layers varies somewhat depending on the method of fixation, and some authors consider the layering to be purely a fixation artefact.

Three types of cell are recognized in the glomerular tuft. *Epithelial* cells envelop the outer surface of the GBM and *endothelial* and *mesangial* cells lie within the GBM. The epithelial cells (or podocytes) are attached to the GBM by innumerable thin cytoplasmic processes (foot processes) (Figure 1.3). Scanning electron microscopy reveals the three-dimensional aspect of their structure and shows that the foot processes form a complex 'herring bone' array, and that the foot processes of adjacent podocytes interdigitate with one another like the clasps of a zip-fastener. High magnification transmission electron microscopy reveals thin diaphragms (slit pore membranes) bridging the gaps between adjacent foot processes (Figure 1.4). It has been suggested that the GBM acts as a 'coarse' filter preventing the escape of large macromolecules from

the vascular compartment, whilst the slit pore membranes act as a fine filter for relatively small macromolecules. The cytoplasm of the tuft epithelial cell contains an abundant granular endoplasmic reticulum, the cisternae of which sometimes contain secretory bodies which may be concerned in the formation of the GBM. The nucleus is characteristically indented and mitochondria are present in its vicinity. Myofilaments and microtubules, arranged randomly or in bundles, are sometimes demonstrable in the foot processes and these may possibly have contractile potential.

Within the confines of the GBM, the endothelial cells line the vascular lumina of the capillaries, and the mesangial cells lie within the stalks of the lobules and are separated from the adjacent capillary lumina by an endothelial cell (Figures 1.5 and 1.6).

The endothelial cell nucleus and much of its cytoplasm is usually situated on the axial side of the capillary loop, but the rest of the capillary circumference is lined by a very thin layer of endothelial cytoplasm. This layer is not completely continuous, being breached at intervals by numerous holes or fenestrations up to 100 nm in diameter. Around the endothelial cell nucleus are mitochondria, a Golgi apparatus and endoplasmic reticulum. Vacuoles of varying size and fibrillar elements are also found in the cytoplasm.

The centrilobular mesangial cells possess numerous cytoplasmic processes which interdigitate between adjacent cells. They are separated by an amorphous fibrillary material (*mesangial matrix*) resembling the GBM in consistency and electron density, and continuous with the lamina rara interna at the edge of the mesangium. Some workers claim that tiny intercellular channels can be demonstrated in the mesangial matrix, and that particulate matter and plasma from the capillary lumina can gain access to them via fenestrations in the endothelial lining of the glomerular capillaries situated over the mesangium. The mesangial cell has an irregularly shaped nucleus with relatively little cytoplasm and the usual organelles. It is presumably responsible for the formation of mesangial matrix, and may be concerned with the regulation of glomerular blood flow. A typical ultrastructural feature is the presence of localized densities on the inner aspect of the cytoplasmic membrane similar to those seen in smooth muscle cell cytoplasm.

Juxtaglomerular Apparatus (Figure 1.7)

The juxtaglomerular apparatus (JGA) is situated at the (vascular) hilum of the glomerulus and has three components:

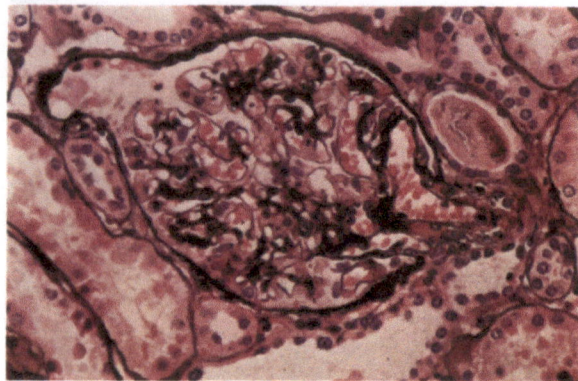

Figure 1.1   A glomerulus stained by Jones' methenamine silver technique to demonstrate normal thickness of mesangial matrix and glomerular capillary basement membranes. × 480.

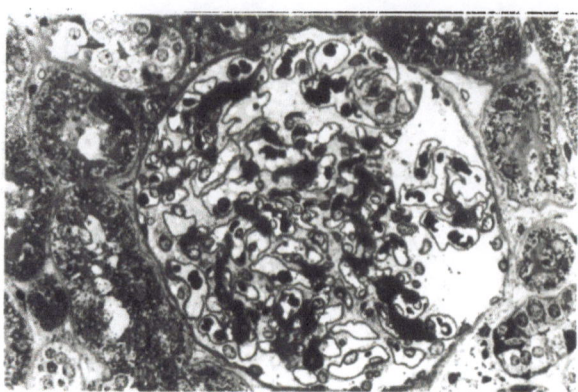

Figure 1.2   A normal glomerulus from a renal biopsy embedded in Epon, and stained with toluidine blue. Note the improved histological clarity achieved by this technique. × 600.

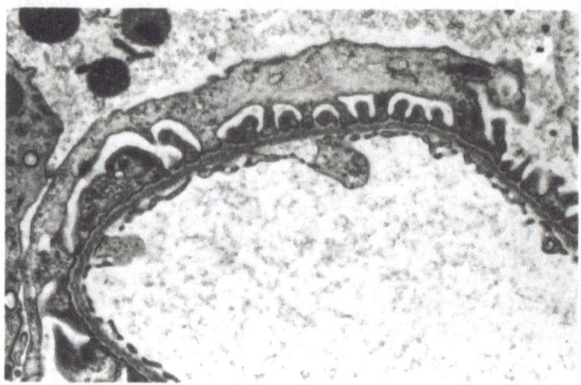

Figure 1.3   Electron microscopy of part of a normal glomerular capillary loop. The basement membrane is composed of a central lamina densa with an inner and outer lamina rara. There is a thin fenestrated lining of endothelial cytoplasm and on the outer aspect of the GBM are the interdigitating foot processes of the epithelial cells. × 7750.

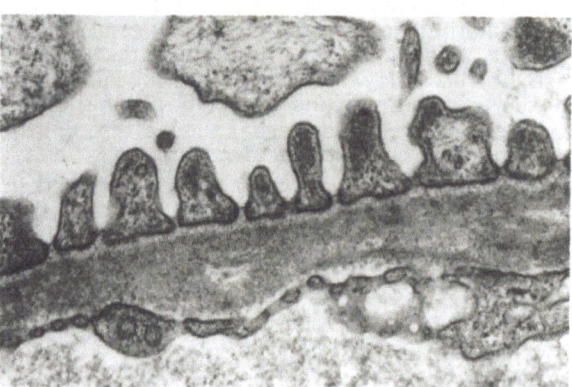

Figure 1.4   High power electron micrograph of GBM showing the thin slit pore membranes between individual epithelial foot processes. × 36 250.

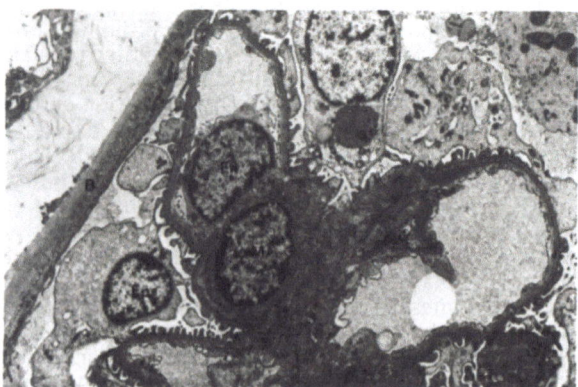

Figure 1.5   Electron micrograph of part of a glomerular tuft lobule. The GBM of the three capillary profiles is continuous. Within its confines are two nuclei: one, that of an endothelial cell (En) lining the capillary lumen, the other, that of a mesangial cell (M). Outside the GBM two epithelial nuclei (Ep) are present together with numerous foot processes. Part of Bowman's capsule (B) is also present with a few collagen fibres. × 3600.

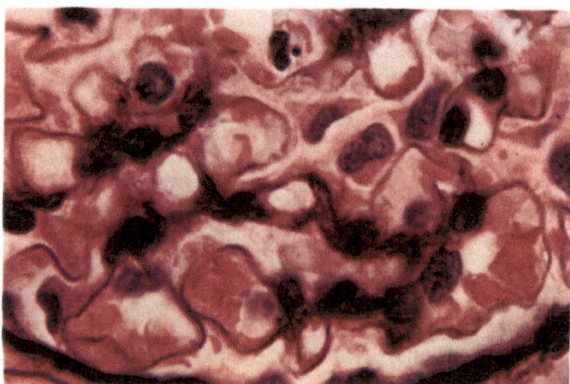

Figure 1.6   High power light photomicrograph of part of a glomerular tuft stained as in Figure 1.1. By comparison with the last figure epithelial, endothelial and mesangial cells can be identified. The capillary lumina contain many red blood cells and a single neutrophil polymorph. The silver impregnation details a normal amount of mesangial matrix. × 1680.

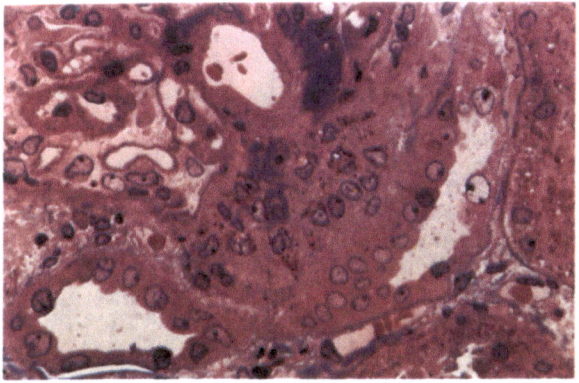

Figure 1.7 The juxtaglomerular apparatus (JGA) is often an incon-spicuous structure unless sectioned fortuitously. This example is hyper-plastic. Towards the top left part of the glomerular tuft an afferent arteriole is visible and in the wall of the latter are many granular epithelioid cells and agranular lacis cells. The distal convoluted tubule is cut across twice and the macula densa is easily recognized by the crowding of the nuclei. × 960.

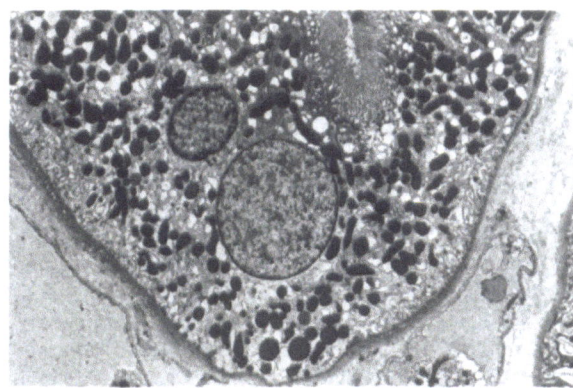

Figure 1.8 An electron micrograph of part of a proximal convoluted tubule showing the microvilli of the brush border and numerous densely staining mitochondria. × 3600.

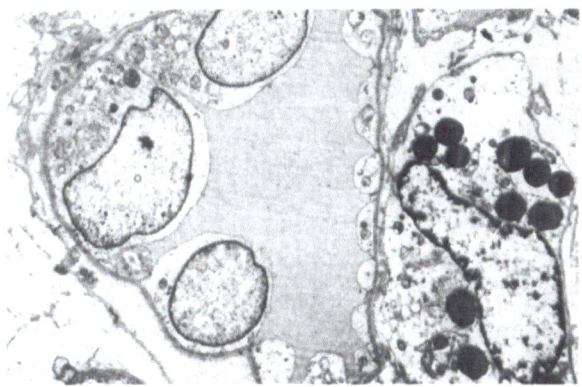

Figure 1.9 Electron micrograph of the thin limb of the loop of Henle (rat kidney). Adjacent to this on the right-hand side is an interstitial cell containing electron-dense lipid droplets. × 4200. (By courtesy of Dr E. A. Molland)

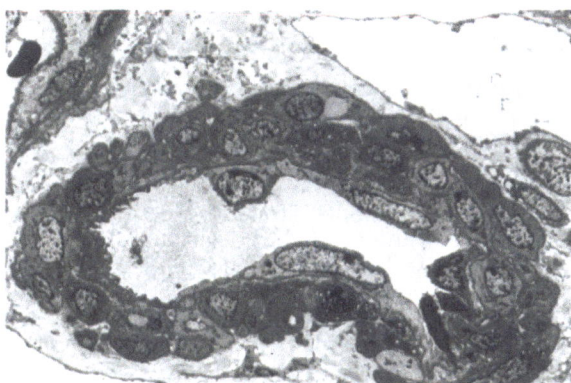

Figure 1.10 Electron micrograph of an afferent arteriole. The wall is composed of smooth muscle cells and the lumen is lined by endothelial cells. Adjacent to the arteriole are thin walled capillaries. × 1625.

(1) Specialized granular epithelioid cells in the wall of the terminal portion of the afferent arteriole,

(2) Modified epithelial cells known collectively as the *macula densa* in the adjacent distal convoluted tubule where it impinges on the vascular pole of the parent glomerulus, and

(3) Agranular cells between the macula densa and the glomerulus called *lacis cells* which ultrastructurally closely resemble glomerular mesangial cells.

The cytoplasmic granules of the epithelioid cells in the afferent arteriole contain a high concentration of renin. The cells of the macula densa probably have a sensory function regulating the release of renin in response to changes in the composition of the tubular fluid in the distal convoluted tubule. Lacis cells may perform a similar regulating function in response to changes in glomerular blood flow.

Proximal Convoluted Tubule (Figure 1.8)

The proximal convoluted tubule forms a tight coil around the glomerulus from which it arises and in histological sections appears as a series of cross-sections surrounding the glomerulus. It is lined by tall cuboidal or columnar epithelial cells resting on a basement membrane (TBM). The cell borders are indistinct and the round vesicular nuclei lie at the bases of the cells near the TBM. The luminal surfaces possess a brush border usually best seen in PAS preparations. Ultrastructurally the brush border is seen to consist of series of microvilli (about 6500/cell) which increase the cellular surface area some 40 times. This segment of the tubule is responsible for selective reabsorption of about 80% of the total solutes and water in the glomerular filtrate, and, as might be expected in such metabolically active cells, large numbers of elongated mitochondria are present. At the bases of the cells the plasma membrane is elaborately infolded and interdigitations occur between adjacent cells. The mitochondria are arranged with their long axes parallel with the long axis of the cell, at right angles to the TBM within the compartments formed by the infolded plasma membrane. Numerous endocytic vesicles are present particularly in the apical part of the cell, and many lysosomes and polyribosomes are present.

Loop of Henle

The thin descending limb and the thin part of the ascending limb are lined by flattened epithelial cells lacking a brush border. Segments of this part of the tubule are best seen in sections of the renal medulla, particularly near the papillary tip, where they lie in close proximity to the vasa recta. Ultrastructurally, the epithelial cells have few surface microvilli and their cytoplasm contains scanty, small mitochondria, a few profiles of endoplasmic reticulum and occasional polyribosomes.

The thick ascending limb is lined by cuboidal cells without brush borders whose nuclei lie nearer the luminal than the basal cell surface. Segments of this portion of the tubule are most clearly identified in the medullary rays as they radiate through the cortex at right angles to the capsular surface. The high

energy requirements of these epithelial cells, which actively pump sodium chloride from the tubular lumen across the cell to the interstitium as part of the countercurrent urinary concentration mechanism, is reflected ultrastructurally by the plentiful elongated mitochondria. These, as in the cells of the proximal convoluted tubules, are arranged perpendicular to the TBM within compartments formed by infolding of the basal plasma membrane. Surface microvilli are scanty and small vesicles are prominent in the apical portions of the cells.

Distal Convoluted Tubule

The distal convoluted tubule is lined by cuboidal epithelium which lacks a brush border. The specialized portion forming the macula densa of the JGA has slightly taller cells in which the nuclei are larger and crowded together. In cross-section under the light microscope, distal convoluted tubules have wider lumina, lower lining epithelial cells and more nuclei per cross-section than proximal convoluted tubules. Ultrastructurally, the distal tubular epithelial cells contain numerous mitochondria which are, however, smaller than those in the proximal tubules. Infolding of the basal plasma membrane is present. Surface microvilli are few and variable numbers of vesicles are present in the apical portions.

Collecting Tubule

The collecting tubules are lined by cuboidal cells with distinct outlines, large central nuclei and pale cytoplasm.

In the rat kidney two types of epithelial cells are recognizable ultrastructurally. These are light (or principal) cells and darker (intercalated) cells in which the cytoplasm is more electron-dense, has more numerous mitochondria and polyribosomes and contains large numbers of apical microvesicles.

Interstitium

In the normal kidney the tubules lie very close together and the interstitium is very sparse, although occasional reticulin fibres can be demonstrated between the tubules by silver staining. In the medulla occasional specialized cells (interstitial cells) lie close to capillaries and the thin limbs of the loops of Henle (Figure 1.9). By electron microscopy these cells can be shown to contain lipid droplets. They are thought to secrete prostaglandins and their possible role in hypertension is of current interest.

Blood Vessels

The intrarenal arteries are muscular in type and have a single internal elastic lamina. The intima consists of little more than a single layer of endothelial cells, but occasionally eccentric cushions of intimal thickening occur where vessels branch.

Interlobar arteries and veins extend radially between the renal papillae in the columns of Bertin. Arcuate vessels lie at the cortico-medullary junction and run in the long axis of the kidney. Interlobular vessels run radially in the cortex and at right angles to the capsule and to the arcuate vessels from which they originate. The interlobular arteries give rise to the afferent arterioles which supply each glomerulus (Figure 1.10).

Congenital Malformations of the Kidney

2

Development of the Kidney

Although transient vestigial excretory organs (the pro- and mesonephros) are recognizable in the human embryo, the definitive kidney is the metanephros. This is formed in two parts: the nephrons from the nephrogenic cord and the excretory ducts (collecting tubules, calyces, pelvis and ureter) from the ureteric bud which grows as a branch from the caudal portion of the mesonephric (Wolffian) duct. During early development the ureteric bud grows cranially and impinges on the caudal end of the nephrogenic cord (called the metanephric blastema) where it begins a process of rapid dichotomous branching. The first few generations of branches coalesce to form the renal pelvis and calyces. As further branching occurs, condensations of metanephric blastema, from which the nephrons develop, become related to the dilated tip, or ampulla, of each branch of the ureteric bud (Figure 2.1). As the nephrons form they become attached to the ampullae which in turn develop into collecting ducts. Attachment to the growing tip of the ureteric bud branches ensures that the nephrons are carried outwards as they develop.

The ways in which the nephrons become attached to the ampulla vary at different stages of organogenesis (Figure 2.2). After the initial phase, branching of the ureteric bud ceases, and each ampulla becomes capable of inducing formation of a number of nephrons which join together in a chain or nephron arcade. After about the 22nd week, in the outer renal cortex, nephrons are attached singly just behind the zone of active ampullary growth until new nephron formation stops at between 32 and 36 weeks of gestation. Individual nephrons form from initially solid, oval condensations of metanephric blastema. These quickly develop a lumen, elongate, become 'S'-shaped and become continuous with the ureteric bud branch. At the distal end a glomerulus develops and the intervening portions form the convoluted tubules and loop of Henle.

Congenital Malformations

Congenital malformations of the kidney and urinary tract are common and when present are associated with malformations in other systems in about 50% of cases.

Developmental anomalies can be classified as follows:

(1) Anomalies of position and form, e.g. ectopia, fusion

(2) Parenchymal anomalies, e.g. agenesis, hypoplasia and dysplasia

(3) Cystic renal disease (see Chapter 3)

Ectopia

Renal ectopia is usually due to failure of cephalic 'migration' of the kidney during development. Most ectopic kidneys are thus located within the pelvis or at the pelvic brim. Normal 'ascent' is accompanied by gradual medial rotation, so that the renal pelvis comes to lie on the medial aspect of the kidney. Ectopic kidneys often fail to rotate so that the renal pelvis lies on their anterior surface. Often, too, they lack a normal reniform shape since they are not subjected to the moulding effect of abdominal viscera normally adjacent to the kidneys. The blood supply of ectopic kidneys is frequently abnormal and the renal arteries may be formed from one or more branches of the aorta near its bifurcation or from the iliac vessels. Renal ectopia may be unilateral or bilateral, and simple (i.e. with the draining ureter on the same side) or crossed (i.e. with the ureter crossing the midline and inserted into the opposite side of the bladder). In unilateral crossed ectopia, the two kidneys are on the same side of the body and may be fused together. The ureter of an ectopic kidney may be inserted ectopically, for example into the urethra or vagina. Parenchymal anomalies, such as renal dysplasia (see below), are commoner in ectopic kidneys, and obstruction of the draining pelvis or ureter leading to hydronephrosis and possibly renal infection is not infrequent.

Fusion

Fusion of the two kidneys across the midline usually occurs at the lower poles producing the so-called 'horseshoe' kidney. Much less commonly both poles are fused (the 'ring' or 'doughnut' kidney).

Renal Agenesis

Complete absence of the kidney may be unilateral or bilateral (Figure 2.3). Bilateral agenesis is incompatible with life and is associated with a syndrome of abnormalities (pulmonary hypoplasia, bow legs, low-set ears, receding chin and a beak-like nose), described by Potter[1] (Figure 2.4). Associated congenital anomalies of the genitalia are common. In the male the testis usually fails to descend and mesonephric duct derivatives such as the vas deferens and seminal vesicle are often absent. In the female paramesonephric duct derivatives (fallopian tubes, uterine horns and upper vagina) are often absent or abnormal. Lower limb anomalies, particularly sirenomelia (posterior limb bud fusion and absence of hind gut, sacrum, bladder, urethra and external genitalia) are frequently accompanied by bilateral renal agenesis.

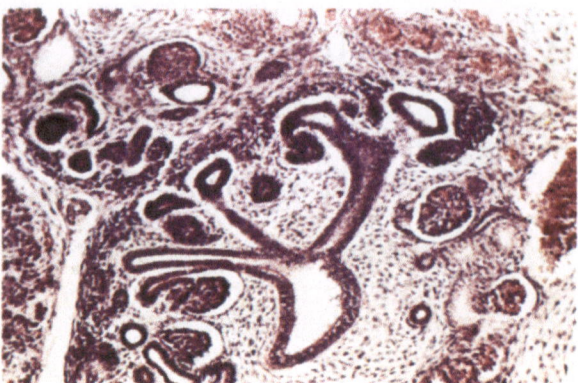

Figure 2.1 A section of renal cortex from a 44 mm human embryo. Dichotomous division of the ureteric bud branches is evident. Their dilated tips (ampullae) are related to condensations of metanephric blastema, from which the nephrons develop. H & E   × 96.

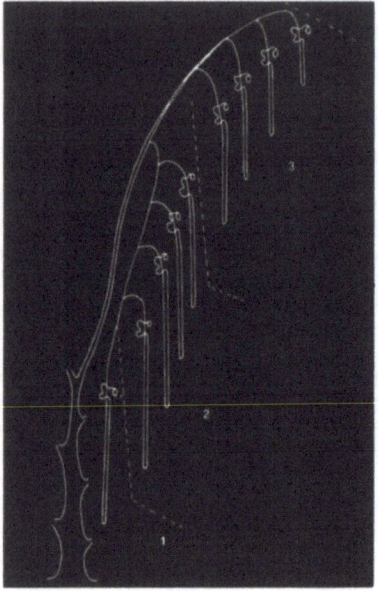

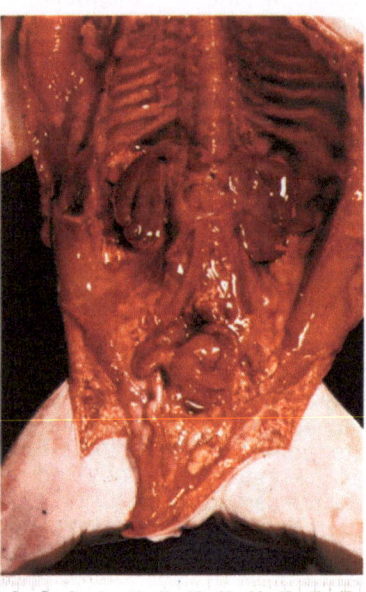

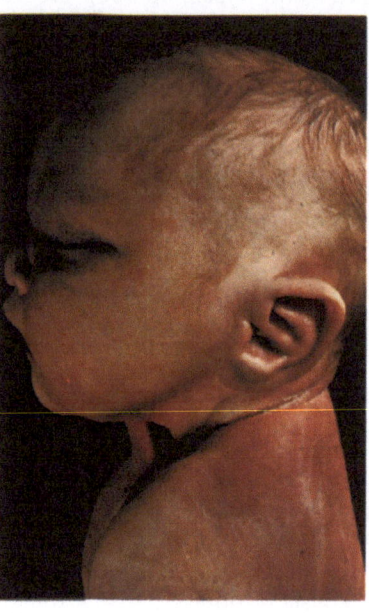

Figure 2.2 Nephron formation[4]; 1 — Nephrons formed during initial phase of ureteric bud branching; 2 — Nephron arcade; 3 — Nephrons adding singly until nephrogenesis ceases at 32–36 weeks.

Figure 2.3 Necropsy appearance of a stillborn infant with bilateral renal agenesis. Note the prominent disc-shaped adrenals (which are occasionally mistaken for small kidneys by the inexperienced) and the associated abnormality of the female genital tract (bicornuate uterus).

Figure 2.4 Side view of the head of the infant shown in Figure 2.3. Note the receding chin, beak-like nose and low-set ears[1].

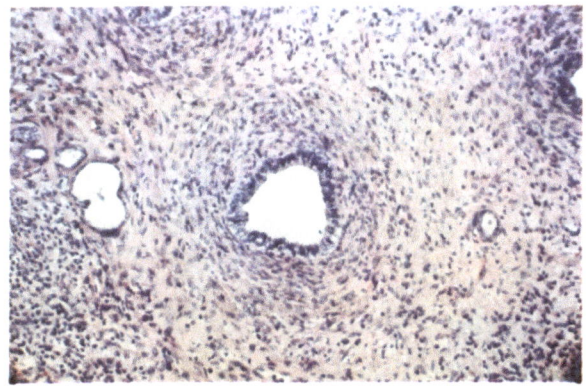

Figure 2.5 Renal dysplasia. A primitive duct lined by columnar epithelium and surrounded by cellular mesenchyme. H & E ×120.

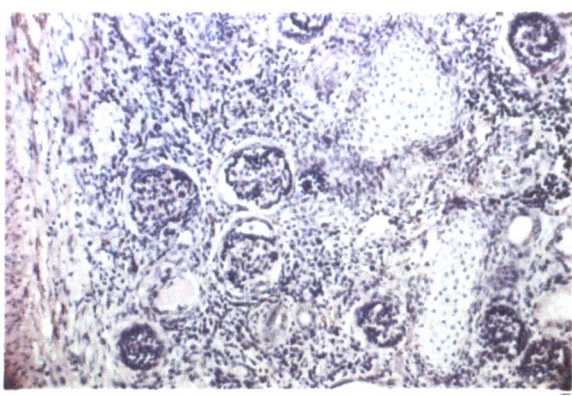

Figure 2.6 Renal dysplasia. An area of cortex showing immature glomeruli and tubules with bars of metaplastic cartilage. H & E ×120.

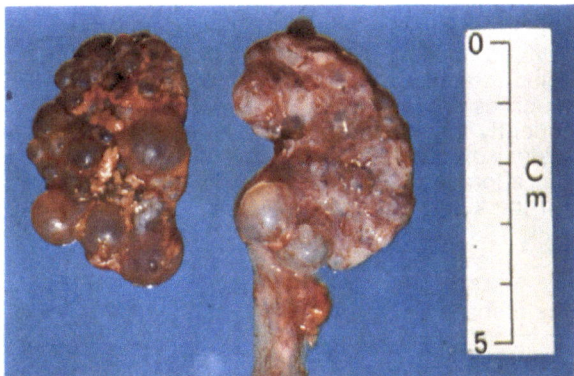

Figure 2.7 Bisected cystic dysplastic kidney. The reniform shape is completely destroyed, the kidney being converted to a multicystic mass.

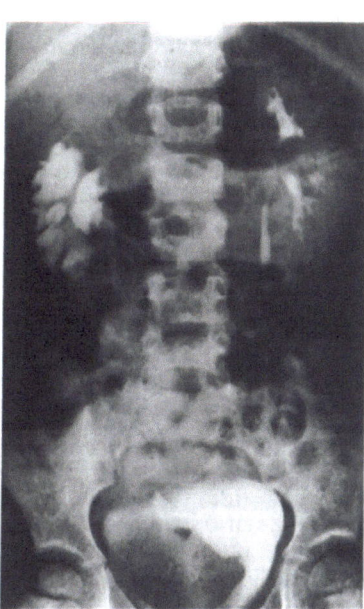

Figure 2.8 Renal tract abnormalities associated with renal dysplasia. An intravenous urogram showing a double (duplex) kidney on the right; the upper pole is dysplastic and fails to excrete contrast medium. The ureter draining this dysplastic upper pole ends in a cystic ureterocoele which produces a filling defect in the bladder, and obstructs the ureter draining the lower pole to produce a degree of pelvicalyceal dilatation (courtesy of the editor of *Pediatric Radiology*).

The normal shape of the adrenal glands is due in part to the effects of moulding by the kidneys. In renal agenesis the adrenals appear disc-shaped and occasionally fail to develop. The corresponding ureter and trigonal area of the bladder are nearly always completely absent in renal agenesis but occasionally a short stump of distal ureter is present. Major anomalies of other systems are common.

Renal Hypoplasia and Dysplasia

Congenitally small (hypoplastic) kidneys are often difficult to diagnose since diminution in renal size may be due to scarring from acquired disease. Conversely hypoplastic kidneys may themselves be prone to acquire lesions such as pyelonephritis, which may mask the underlying congenital anomaly.

The majority of congenitally small kidneys show evidence of anomalous metanephric differentiation on microscopical examination and such kidneys are termed dysplastic. The term renal hypoplasia is preserved for kidneys whose developmental abnormality lies only in their diminished size, and perhaps in their reduced numbers of lobules (reniculi).

Simple hypoplasia without dysplasia is very rare and nearly always bilateral. The most extreme examples of bilateral renal hypoplasia are encountered in *oligomeganephronie* (oligonephronic hypoplasia). The kidneys are extremely small (often with combined weights of less than 20 g), and are composed of only one or two lobules. The number of nephrons present is severely reduced, but those present are often enormously hypertrophied[2].

Renal dysplasia is a form of hypoplasia in which evidence of metanephric maldifferentiation is apparent on histology. The microscopic changes include disorganization of the renal parenchyma, the presence of immature nephronic and ductal structures normally encountered only in the fetal kidney, and sometimes cyst formation. The most important findings from a diagnostic view point are the presence of *primitive ducts* and bars of *metaplastic cartilage* (Figures 2.5 and 2.6). Primitive ducts are tubular structures, often occurring in nodular aggregates which are lined by columnar or ciliated epithelium, and surrounded by concentric mantles of cellular mesenchyme in which smooth muscle cells can occasionally be identified. These ducts are

regarded as persisting branches of the ureteric bud which they closely resemble. Bars of metaplastic cartilage are found most frequently in the outer subcapsular regions and are thought to be the result of aberrant differentiation of metanephric blastema. Primitive ducts are the *sine qua non* of renal dysplasia and this histological diagnosis should not be made in their absence. Metaplastic cartilage is by no means invariable but is useful confirmatory evidence of dysplasia.

Dysplastic alteration may be focal, segmental or involve the whole kidney. Affected kidneys are generally smaller than normal, but if cyst formation is marked they may be grossly enlarged, even though the actual amount of parenchyma is reduced (Figure 2.7).

An important diagnostic feature of renal dysplasia is the frequent association with other congenital anomalies of the ureter or lower urinary tract[3]. Such abnormalities are usually obstructive or associated with vesico-ureteric reflux (Figure 2.8). The presence of obstruction at an early stage of renal development probably accounts for the altered metanephric differentiation of renal dysplasia, and also explains why acquired diseases such as pyelonephritis or hydronephrosis may frequently be superimposed on dysplastic kidneys. Renal dysplasia is thus more logically regarded as an anomaly of the whole urinary tract rather than of the kidney alone.

References

1. Potter, E. L. (1946). Facial characteristics of infants with bilateral renal agenesis. *Am. J. Obstet. Gynecol.*, **51**, 885–888.

2. Royer, P., Habib, R., Mathieu, H. and Courtecuisse, V. (1962). L'hypoplasie rénale bilaterale congénital avec reduction du nombre et hypertrophie des nephrons chez l'enfant. *Ann. Pediatr.*, **9**, 133–146.

3. Risdon, R. A. (1971). Renal dysplasia. Part I. A clinicopathological study of 76 cases. Part II. A necropsy study of 41 cases. *J. Clin. Pathol.*, **24**, 57–71.

4. Osathanondh, V. and Potter, E. L. (1963 and 1966). Development of human kidneys as shown by microdissection. A series of five articles: *Arch. Pathol.*, **76**, 271–276, 277–289, 290–302; **82**, 391–402, 403–411.

Renal cysts, particularly when they are multiple, tend to be regarded as developmental anomalies. It is important to recognize, however, that many renal cysts are acquired lesions. One or more renal cysts can be found at necropsy in about half of all subjects over 50 years of age, and their comparative rarity in children and young adults strongly supports their acquired nature. These 'simple' cysts appear to arise by local blockage of nephrons by focal scarring and they are particularly common in arteriosclerotic kidneys. Occasionally very extensive cystic transformation is encountered in the chronically diseased kidneys of patients maintained on longterm renal dialysis[1] and this provides a further striking example of acquired renal cystic disease. Renal cysts are, however, a prominent feature of a number of developmental disorders which can be defined by their clinical presentations and special pathological features. Cystic forms of renal dysplasia (Chapter 2) are important examples. Some varieties of developmental renal cysts are heritable and their accurate diagnosis is important for genetic counselling.

Polycystic Disease

This term has been applied loosely to any kidney with multiple cysts, whether developmental or acquired, and this has lead to considerable confusion. There are two varieties of cystic disease to which the name polycystic disease is given correctly.

'Adult' Polycystic Disease

Clinical recognition of patients with this condition is usually delayed until adult life, most frequently in the fourth decade. The most common presentation is chronic renal failure, usually accompanied by hypertension; occasionally haematuria is noted. Although not common, the disease is well within the experience of most pathologists. It is inherited as an autosomal dominant trait, but about 50% of cases result from a new mutation so that a previous family history may not be obtained.

Macroscopically, cysts of varying size are present throughout both kidneys which at the time of diagnosis are usually enlarged (sometimes weighing more than 1000 grams) and have lost their reniform shape (Figure 3.1). The cysts arise in any part of the nephron or collecting system and tend to distort the pelvi-calyceal system, a change which can be identified radiologically at a pre-symptomatic stage. Haemorrhage into the cysts may cause loin pain or haematuria and renal infection may occur, particularly terminally. Cysts are often found in other organs such as the liver (Figure 3.6), pancreas and lung,

but rarely give rise to symptoms. Berry aneurysm of the cerebral vessels is another association and subarachnoid haemorrhage from rupture of such aneurysms is the cause of death in about 10% of cases.

The relatively uncommon cases diagnosed in childhood or early adult life usually exhibit less extensive cyst formation, and it seems probable that the cysts develop gradually in initially normal nephtons and collecting ducts (Figure 3.2). It is only when sufficient parenchyma has been rendered cystic or has been destroyed by pressure from adjacent cysts that renal function becomes impaired. The autosomal dominant inheritance of the condition has led to the suggestion by Darmady et al.[2] that cyst formation is caused by excretion of an unidentified abnormal metabolite produced by a genetically determined enzyme defect. It has been noted, however, that cystic disease does not develop in renal allografts transplanted into patients with this condition, although the time scale in which this could develop is much shorter.

'Infantile' Polycystic Disease

This is much rarer than the adult variety. Classically it is seen in stillbirths or in infants who die in the neonatal period, and family studies indicate an autosomal recessive mode of inheritance. Both kidneys are enlarged, sometimes many times the normal size, but they retain their reniform shape and display accentuated fetal lobulation (Figure 3.3). The pelvicalyceal system is normal and the renal parenchyma is replaced by radially orientated, fusiform or cylindrical cysts throughout both cortex and medulla (Figure 3.7). Histologically the cysts are seen as dilatations of the collecting ducts. The glomeruli are normal but are widely separated from each other by the intervening cysts; the overall number of nephrons and glomeruli is not reduced. Interstitial fibrosis is not a conspicuous feature (Figure 3.4).

In every case of infantile polycystic disease an hepatic abnormality is present (Figure 3.8). This consists of proliferation and angulated branching of bile ducts in every portal tract[3]. This is associated with a variable degree of portal fibrosis and is termed congenital hepatic fibrosis (Figure 3.9).

The association between renal cystic disease and congenital hepatic fibrosis is incompletely understood. Whilst the classical form of infantile polycystic disease is invariably accompanied by the hepatic anomaly, congenital hepatic fibrosis may also occur with lesser degrees of renal cystic disease and even in its absence. In some examples with renal cystic disease, renal function may be only moderately or slightly impaired, or even normal. The

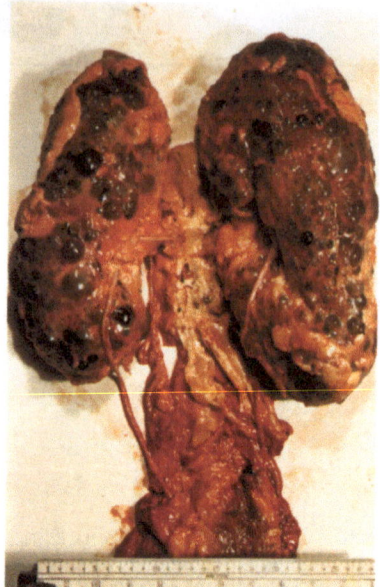

Figure 3.1 'Adult' polycystic disease in a middle-aged man. The cysts which vary in size are scattered diffusely throughout the parenchyma and distort the renal outline. Some cysts are dark due to altered blood within their cavities.

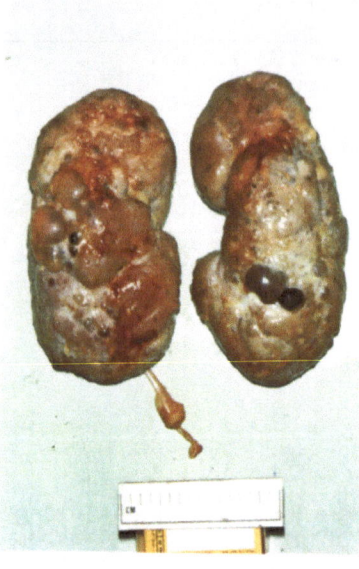

Figure 3.2 'Adult' polycystic kidneys from an 11-year-old child dying with sub-arachnoid haemorrhage from a ruptured berry aneurysm. Comparing the kidneys in this young patient with those in Figure 3.1, it is evident that the extent of cyst formation is considerably less marked.

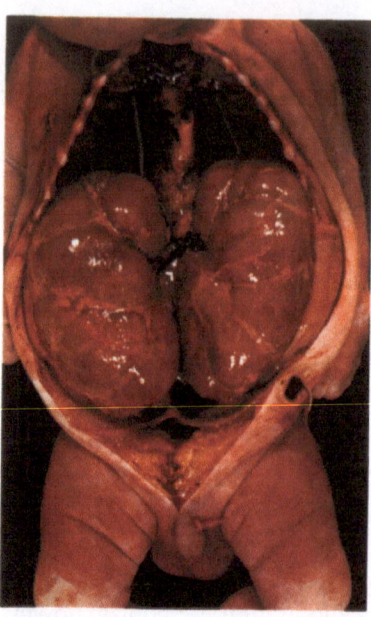

Figure 3.3 Necropsy appearance of a male neonate dying from 'infantile' polycystic disease. Note the huge size of the kidneys which nevertheless retain their reniform shape and show exaggerated fetal lobulation.

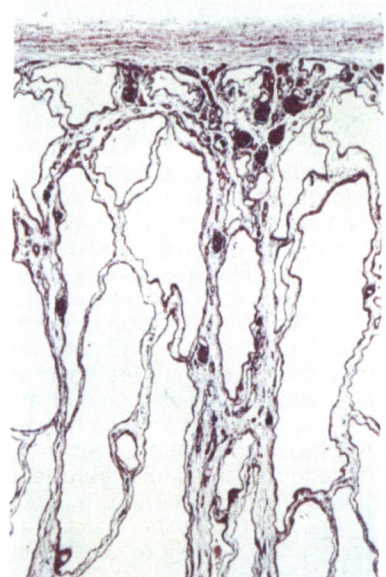

Figure 3.4 Low power photomicrograph of the sub-capsular cortex in 'infantile' polycystic disease showing that the cysts are largely derived from grossly dilated collecting ducts. H & E × 30.

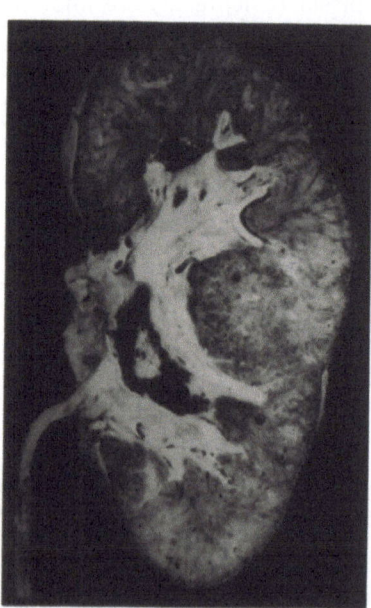

Figure 3.5 Kidney from a 10-year-old child with juvenile nephronophthisis. The kidney is about half the expected size and is diffusely contracted, there being no localized scar formation (a useful distinction from the kidney of reflux nephropathy). Scattered tiny cysts mainly near the cortico-medullary junction are visible on the cut surface. Kidney photographed with UV light to enhance surface detail (courtesy of the editor of *Pediatric Radiology*).

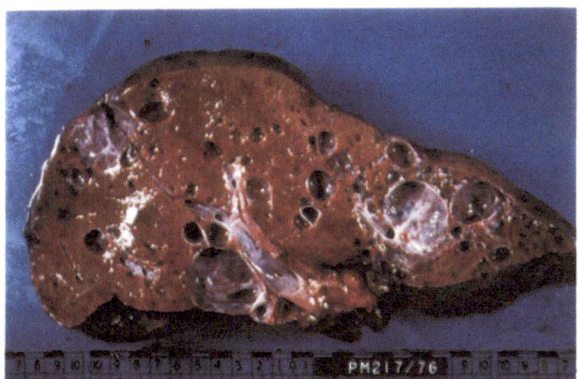

Figure 3.6 The liver from a patient with 'adult' polycystic disease; the cut surface is studded with cysts of variable size having thin walls and smooth epithelial linings. Some degree of cystic change is present in the liver in about 30% of these patients, who nevertheless have normal hepatic function.

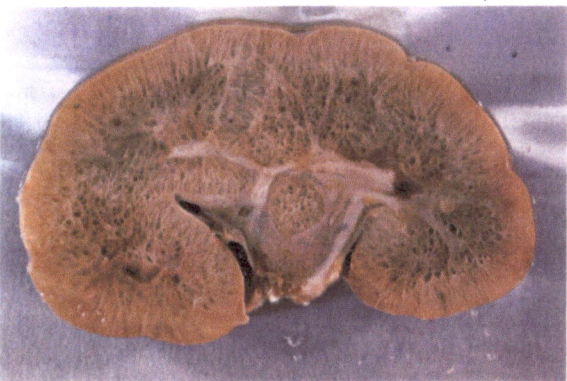

Figure 3.7 Cut surface of the kidney in 'infantile' polycystic disease showing the retention of cortico-medullary demarcation and the transformation of the parenchyma by innumerable radially aligned fusiform cysts.

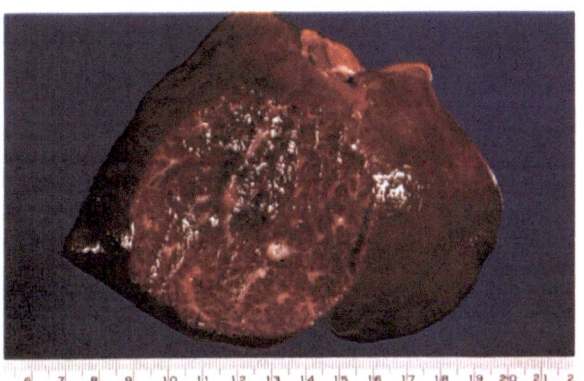

Figure 3.8 The liver from an infant with 'infantile' polycystic disease showing changes of congenital hepatic fibrosis, i.e. an obvious increase in fibrous connective tissue in portal tracts.

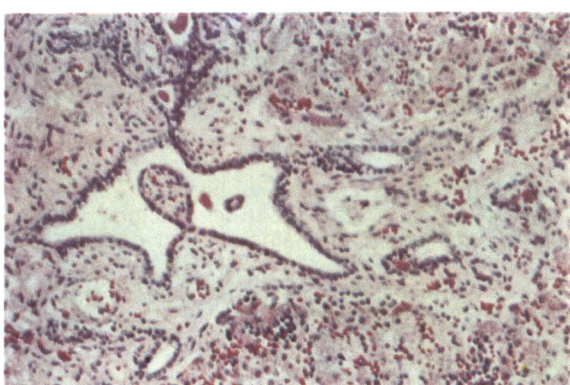

Figure 3.9 Photomicrograph of a portal tract within the liver in 'infantile' polycystic disease showing an increase in connective tissue and the curious proliferation and angulated branching of bile ducts which often appear to run in the plane of section. Serial reconstructions suggest that these bile channels form a series of interconnected cisterns rather than tubular ducts[3] H & E × 360.

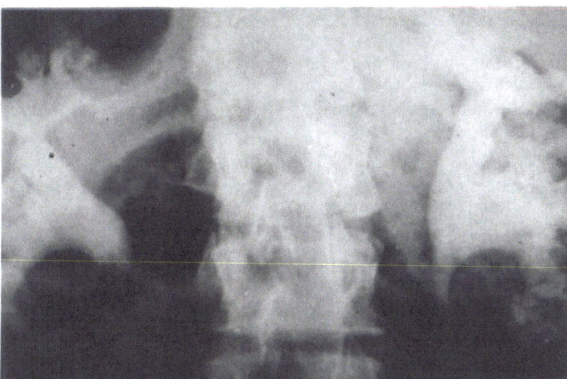

Figure 3.10 An intravenous urogram in a patient with medullary sponge kidney. Ectasia of the medullary collecting ducts is particularly prominent in the left lower pole.

cystic transformation may affect only some of the collecting ducts or may be confined to the papillary ducts.

Whilst infants with the classical form of infantile polycystic disease are anuric and either are stillborn or die in the neonatal period, it is increasingly recognized that a minority of infants with this disease survive into childhood or even to adult life with varying degrees of renal impairment. Such individuals are likely to be those with lesser degrees of renal cystic disease. In those patients whose renal disease is less serious, however, there is a tendency for the hepatic lesion to progress. Increasing portal fibrosis ultimately leads to portal hypertension and the clinical presentation is then likely to be bleeding from oesophageal varices. Infantile polycystic disease and congenital hepatic fibrosis thus form a continuous spectrum. Blyth and Ockenden[4] have shown that, while inheritance is autosomal recessive in type, within a particular family the relative degrees of renal and hepatic involvement tend to breed true and on this basis they suggest that a number of different mutant genes may be responsible.

A further complication is that the lesion of congenital hepatic fibrosis also occurs in association with other very rare familial forms of renal cystic disease, notably Meckel's syndrome. This is an autosomal recessive condition in which congenital hepatic fibrosis accompanies bilateral multicystic renal dysplasia. Other features include microcephaly, posterior encephalocoele, polydactyly, cleft palate and genital anomalies.

Medullary Cystic Disease

Medullary Sponge Kidney

This is a radiological rather than a pathological entity in which intravenous urography demonstrates dilated medullary collecting ducts (so-called 'ductal ectasia') (Figure 3.10). Flecks of medullary calcification may also be visible. The kidneys are either slightly enlarged or of normal size. This entity is often an incidental finding since the patients are often asymptomatic with normal renal function. Occasionally stone formation or urinary tract infection may bring the condition to light. The diagnosis is usually made in adult life and only rarely in childhood. A family history is very unusual and associated abnormalities are rare, although occasionally hemihypertrophy is noted. Renal involvement may be unilateral or bilateral.

It should be emphasized that exactly similar radiological appearances may be obtained in rare examples of infantile polycystic disease where cyst formation is confined to the medulla. Such cases may be distinguished by the accompanying congenital hepatic fibrosis. The pathology of the medullary sponge kidney is, as yet, incompletely characterized since it is rare that a full pathological examination is possible.

Medullary Cystic Disease (Juvenile Nephronophthisis)

Medullary cystic disease and juvenile nephronophthisis were first described separately[5, 6], the former characterized pathologically by the presence of prominent cysts at the cortico-medullary junction, and the latter as a form of hereditary nephropathy causing polyuria and renal failure in children (Figure 3.5).

The pathology of both is similar with severe cortical changes comprising extensive glomerulosclerosis, tubular loss and atrophy, and focal interstitial chronic inflammation. The only distinction is the presence of macroscopic cystic change most prominent at the cortico-medullary junction in medullary cystic disease. This is probably insufficient evidence that the two conditions are distinct since the clinical features are often identical and cases with and without medullary cysts have been described in the same sibship. The spectrum of medullary cystic disease/juvenile nephronophthisis is not completely homogeneous, however, and in particular there is evidence of genetic heterogenicity. Cases presenting in childhood show an apparent autosomal recessive type of inheritance, whilst those first seen in adult life appear either sporadically or have an autosomal dominant inheritance. Some cases are associated with extrarenal anomalies, usually pigmentary degeneration of the retina and cataracts, and these examples usually show an autosomal recessive inheritance.

Cases presenting in childhood, and by common usage generally described as having juvenile nephronophthisis, have a characteristic clinical picture. Symptoms include thirst, polyuria, polydipsia, nocturia and salt craving. Growth retardation is marked and progressive renal failure develops usually causing death about the end of the first decade without dialysis or renal transplantation. A normocytic normochromic anaemia disproportionate to the degree of renal failure is often a feature. The urine is dilute, proteinuria is trivial or absent and no excess of cells is seen. Urinary salt wasting is characteristic and signs of renal osteodystrophy usually develop with advancing renal failure. In adults the clinical picture is of a salt wasting syndrome resembling Addison's disease but unresponsive to mineralocorticoid therapy.

References

1. Dunnill, M. S., Millard, P. R. and Oliver, D. (1977). Acquired cystic disease of the kidneys: a hazard of long-term intermittent maintenance haemodialysis. *J. Clin. Pathol.*, **30**, 868–877.

2. Darmady, E. M., Offer, J. and Woodhouse, M. A. (1970). Toxic metabolic defect in polycystic disease of kidney. *Lancet*, **1**, 547–550.

3. Jørgensen, M. (1972). Three-dimensional reconstruction of intrahepatic bile ducts in a case of polycystic disease of the liver in an infant. *Acta Pathol. Microbiol. Scand. Section A*, **80**, 201–206.

4. Blyth, H. and Ockenden, B. G. (1971). Polycystic disease of the kidney and liver presenting in childhood. *J. Med. Genet.*, **8**, 257–284.

5. Smith, C. H. and Graham, J. B. (1945). Congenital medullary cysts of the kidneys with severe refractory anaemia. *Am. J. Dis. Child.*, **69**, 369–377.

6. Fanconi, G., Hanhart, E., von Albertini, A., Euhlinger, R., Dohvo, E. and Prader, A. (1951). Die Familiäre juvenile nephronophthise. *Helv. Paediatr. Acta*, **6**, 1–49.

Renal Infection

4

Pyelonephritis is defined as bacterial infection of the kidney and upper urinary tract. Both acute and chronic forms occur and are often accompanied by urinary tract obstruction which is itself associated with a twenty-fold increased incidence of pyelonephritis.

Infection may reach the kidney via the blood stream or by ascent from the lower urinary tract. Ascending infection is usually deemed the more important mechanism and indeed prior infection of the lower tract is frequent. Vesico-ureteric reflux is the most important cause of ascending infection, particularly during infancy and childhood. Bloodstream spread to the kidney is probably underemphasized. Transient bacteraemia certainly occurs with lower tract infections, and renal localization of blood-borne organisms may be encouraged by urinary obstruction. Haematogenous transmission of Gram-negative organisms to the kidney is recognized as an occasional complication of urethral instrumentation.

Acute Pyelonephritis

Pathological descriptions of acute pyelonephritis usually relate to severe bilateral fulminating infections seen at necropsy. These are generally associated with urinary obstruction (caused by prostatic enlargement, tumours of the bladder and cervix, urolithiasis, congenital anomalies etc.) or are part of a generalized septicaemia (the so-called 'pyaemic' kidney).

Macroscopically the kidneys are swollen; small abscesses are scattered beneath the capsule and throughout the parenchyma. The bulging cut surface is marked by blotchy linear and wedge-shaped areas of pallor and congestion (Figure 4.1). The pelvi-calyceal system is dilated where there is urinary obstruction and the lining mucosa is congested, oedematous and usually covered by purulent exudate. Some or all of the renal papillae may be yellow and necrotic and demarcated by a haemorrhagic rim (necrotizing papillitis). This particular complication usually occurs in elderly patients with urinary obstruction or diabetes mellitus. Microscopically, areas of affected cortex show widespread suppurative inflammation; the oedematous interstitium shows a diffuse, dense mixed inflammatory cell infiltrate often with focal abscess formation (Figure 4.2). The interstitial inflammatory cell infiltrate contains numerous polymorphonuclear leukocytes and these predominate in the abscesses. Usually by the time histological examination is made, however, a variable number of chronic inflammatory cells, particularly plasma cells, are also present and in many areas may be the principal cell

type. The rapidity at which the nature of the inflammatory response in acute pyelonephritis changes from an acute pyogenic to an active chronic reaction has been confirmed by experimental observations where the transformation occurs in only a few days[1]. Polymorphs are also frequently seen within surviving tubules and collecting ducts. Tubular destruction may be marked, although glomeruli and blood vessels are on the whole remarkably well preserved. Occasional glomeruli, particularly those within areas of severe inflammation, may exhibit partial tuft necrosis, neutrophil infiltration or focal fibrin deposition. Similarly occasional small blood vessels may show inflammatory destruction of their walls.

It is important to recognize that the severe changes described above may not be typical of the milder upper tract infections seen clinically, in which urinary infection is accompanied by symptoms such as loin pain. Such infections may be largely confined to the ureter and renal pelvis (acute pyelitis) and any parenchymal involvement may be very mild and focally distributed[2]. It is particularly in such cases that renal biopsy with its substantial sampling error is an inappropriate aid to diagnosis. The presence of pus cells within tubules is not infrequently found at necropsy in the scarred kidneys of patients dying with chronic glomerulonephritis, diabetic glomerulosclerosis, cystic kidneys etc. If this does represent renal parenchymal infection complicating other chronic renal diseases then it is probably the result of a terminal bacteraemia.

Chronic Pyelonephritis

This can be regarded as the end result of bacterial infection of the kidney. Pathologically it can be usefully divided into obstructive and non-obstructive forms. In the *obstructive type* – where overt obstruction can be demonstrated in the draining ureter or lower urinary tract – the pelvis and calyces are dilated and the renal parenchyma is uniformly reduced in thickness. Histological examination shows a combination of obstructive atrophy and chronic inflammation which may be focal or diffuse. There is considerable interstitial fibrosis accompanied by tubular atrophy and loss (Figure 4.3). Sometimes aggregates of atrophic tubules filled with homogeneous eosinophilic material give a 'thyroid-like' appearance (Figure 4.4). Interstitial chronic inflammation is characterized by lymphocytic infiltration, usually with an admixture of plasma cells and histiocytes; well-formed lymphoid follicles are often present both in the renal interstitium and beneath the epithelium lining the renal pelvis (Figure 4.5). Glomerular changes are variable; in extensively

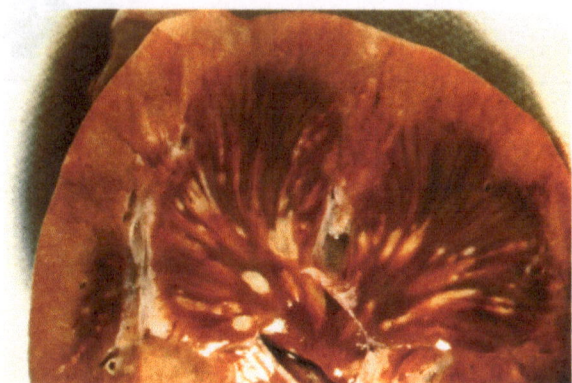

Figure 4.1 Acute pyelonephritis. Cut surface of the kidney illustrating blotchy areas of yellowish-grey pallor and yellow–white linear streaks in the medulla corresponding to polymorph accumulations in collecting tubules and surrounding interstitium.

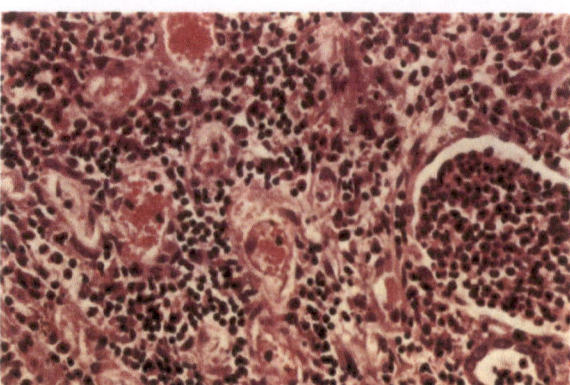

Figure 4.2 Acute pyelonephritis. There is tubular destruction, active chronic inflammatory cell infiltration of the interstitium and a dilated collecting duct filled with neutrophil polymorphs. H & E × 600.

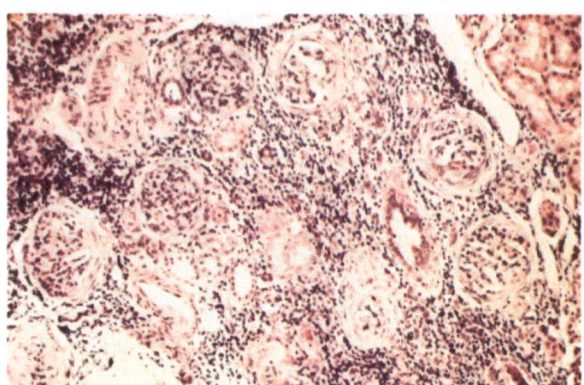

Figure 4.3 Chronic pyelonephritis. Renal cortex showing crowding of glomeruli due to loss of intervening tubules, interstitial chronic inflammation, peri-glomerular fibrosis and focal glomerular scarring H & E. × 120.

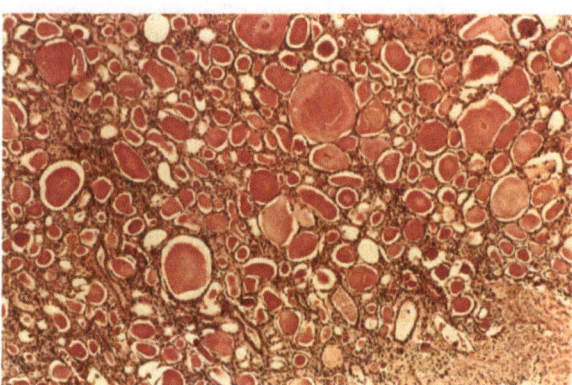

Figure 4.4 Chronic pyelonephritis. Thyroid-like appearance of protein casts in dilated atrophic tubules. This appearance is common in chronic pyelonephritis but is entirely non-specific. H & E × 120.

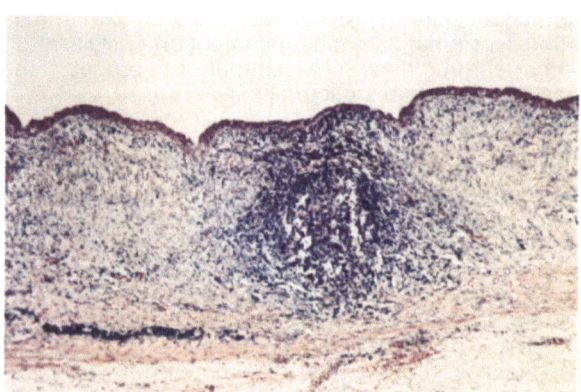

Figure 4.5 Chronic pyelonephritis. Chronic inflammation with lymphoid follicle formation beneath the epithelium of the renal pelvis. H & E × 60.

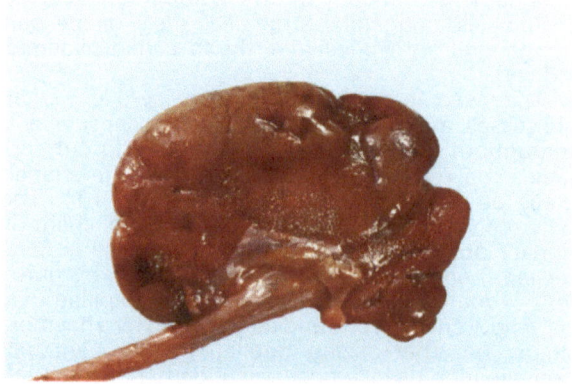

Figure 4.6 Non-obstructive chronic pyelonephritis (reflux nephropathy). The kidney from a child with a history of vesico-ureteric reflux and recurrent urinary tract infection. The kidney is small (50 grams), scarring is segmental and most marked at the poles.

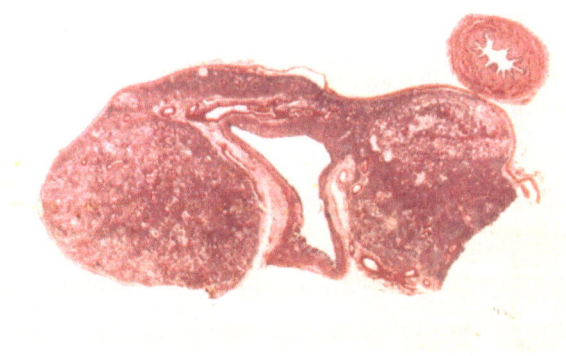

Figure 4.7 Chronic pyelonephritis. The segmental scar is situated directly over a dilated ('clubbed') calyx and its margin is sharply demarcated from the surrounding normal parenchyma. H & E ×2.4.

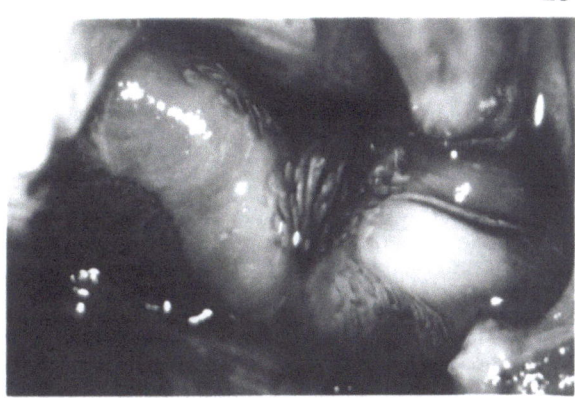

Figure 4.8 Large compound papilla (pig). The area cribrosa is indented and the papillary duct orifices are wide open. They cannot be occluded by a rise in intracalyceal pressure and therefore allow free intrarenal reflux. Papillae of this type occur predominantly at the poles of the kidney where segmental scarring in reflux nephropathy is most common. (Courtesy of the editor of *British Journal of Radiology*.)

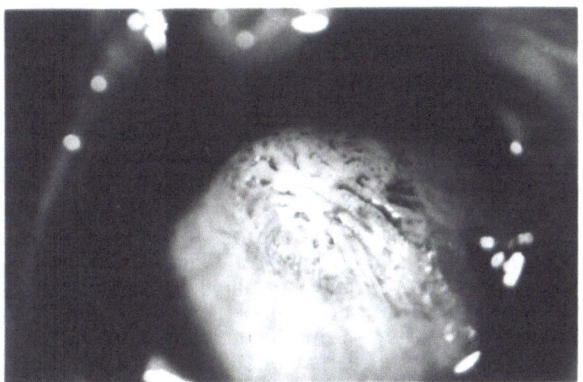

Figure 4.9 Simple conical papilla (pig). The papillary duct orifices are slit-like and tend to close when the intracalyceal pressure rises during vesicoureteric reflux. Intrarenal reflux does not therefore occur. This type of papilla is most numerous in the mid-zone of the kidney where scarring is less common in reflux nephropathy. (Courtesy of the editor of *British Journal of Radiology*.)

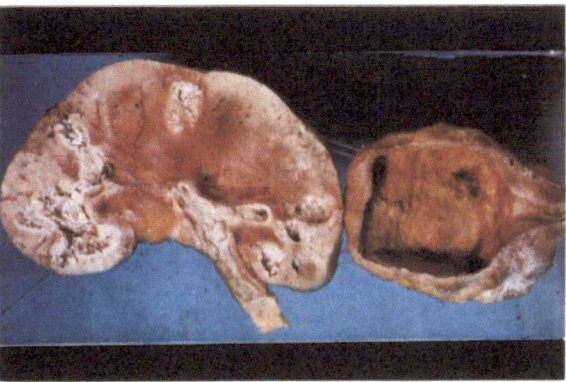

Figure 4.10 Renal tuberculosis. The tuberculous cavities communicate with the pelvicalyceal system. They are lined by caseous material with considerable surrounding fibrosis and often calcification, which gradually destroys the parenchyma. Involvement of the renal pelvis may lead to stricture formation and tuberculous pyonephrosis. Renal tuberculosis may involve part or all of the kidney and associated tuberculous cystitis is almost invariable.

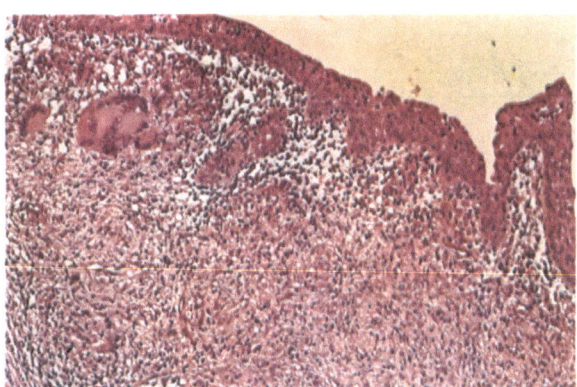

Figure 4.11 Renal tuberculosis. Granulomatous inflammation with multinucleate giant cell formation beneath the urothelium of the renal pelvis. H & E ×120.

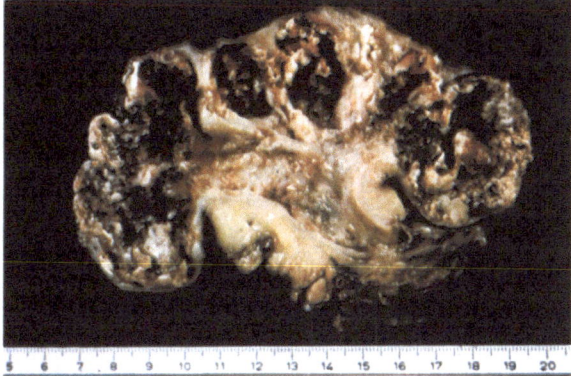

Figure 4.12 Xanthogranulomatous pyelonephritis. The papillae are largely destroyed and the pelvicalyceal system is dilated and surrounded by a yellow zone. This is due to large numbers of lipid-laden macrophages. This type of reaction is often associated with 'stag horn' calculi and *Proteus sp* is the most common infecting organism. Perirenal fibrosis and adhesions may cause technical difficulties when surgical removal is attempted and may lead to a mistaken diagnosis of renal carcinoma.

scarred areas the glomeruli may appear crowded together as a result of tubular loss and interstitial fibrosis. A proportion of glomeruli is completely destroyed and converted to virtually acellular rounded scars. Others are relatively normal or show 'ischaemic' changes (see page 27) which may include segmental sclerosis. Often glomeruli are surrounded by rims of peri-glomerular fibrosis. Vascular changes, such as arterial fibroelastic intimal hyperplasia, are often marked even in the absence of hypertension.

Long-standing urinary obstruction may produce extreme parenchymal thinning, the renal substance being reduced to an attenuated rim of largely collagenous tissue in which only a few scarred glomeruli and atrophic tubules, together with meshes of tortuous, thick-walled blood vessels, can be recognized. Scattered foci of chronic inflammatory cells are present in the interstitium and in the subepithelial tissues around the dilated calyces, pelvis and ureter. Chronic inflammatory changes in the mucosa of the collecting system may be useful in distinguishing renal infection from other types of interstitial nephritis.

In some cases of obstructive pyelonephritis, numerous lipid-filled macrophages accumulate in the renal interstitium. This is referred to as xanthogranulomatous pyelonephritis (Figure 4.12).

Non-obstructive chronic pyelonephritis (so-called because no overt obstruction is demonstrable in the draining ureter or lower urinary tract) is increasingly recognized as a cause of chronic renal failure and/or hypertension in children. Characteristically the kidney is smaller than expected with coarse segmental scars which lie directly over dilated ('clubbed') calyces (Figures 4.6 and 4.7). Usually the scars and calyceal clubbing affect only part of the kidney (principally the polar regions) and occasionally only a single system is involved. The disease may be confined to one kidney but is usually bilateral. The parenchymal scars tend to be wedge-shaped and fairly sharply demarcated from adjacent normal parenchyma. Histological changes within the scars resemble closely those seen in the obstructive form.

It is increasingly apparent that the non-obstructive chronic pyelonephritis seen principally in childhood is the result of vesico-ureteric reflux and the term 'reflux nephropathy' is now frequently used to describe it. Vesico-ureteric reflux means the retrograde propulsion of urine up the ureter from the bladder during micturition. It results from an abnormality of the vesico-ureteric junction which may be primary or be associated with other congenital anomalies. Both clinical and experimental observations[3–5] relate the segmental renal scarring to an extension of vesico-ureteric reflux from the renal pelvis into the tubular system of the kidney (intrarenal reflux). This provides a mechanism whereby any pathogenic organisms present in the urine can gain access to the renal parenchyma. It has also been suggested that the hydrodynamic effects of intrarenal reflux may cause scarring even in the absence of infection. The predominantly polar distribution of scars can be related to papillary morphology (Figures 4.8 and 4.9).

Although reflux nephropathy in its simplest form and in the presence of a history of vesico-ureteric reflux is easily recognized, reflux and obstruction can co-exist and long-standing severe vesico-ureteric reflux may produce hydronephrotic changes in the kidney like those seen in obstruction. In either event the distinction between changes of obstructive and non-obstructive chronic pyelonephritis become blurred. In addition, segmental renal scarring, particularly in older children or young adults in whom vesico-ureteric reflux is not demonstrable may nevertheless be due to reflux nephropathy. Current clinical and experimental evidence strongly suggests that renal scarring occurs early, probably in infancy. Furthermore there is a tendency for vesico-ureteric reflux to cease spontaneously with the passage of time in a proportion of affected children so that it may not be demonstrable in a patient presenting with renal scarring in later childhood. Some of these cases are investigated for arterial hypertension and have been diagnosed as 'segmental renal hypoplasia' (the Ask–Upmark kidney). Currently there is doubt that segmental hypoplasia is a separate entity from reflux nephropathy, since vesico-ureteric reflux is present or has been previously demonstrated in quite a proportion of these cases. It has been recognized recently[6, 7] that late deterioration in renal function, usually accompanied by significant proteinuria, in patients with reflux nephropathy may be associated with glomerular lesions outside the scarred areas which resemble morphologically the changes seen in focal glomerulosclerosis and hyalinosis (see page 59).

Renal Tuberculosis

Tuberculous involvement of the kidney is invariably blood-borne usually from an initial lesion in the lungs. Sometimes the pulmonary lesions heal before the renal infection becomes clinically apparent (so-called isolated organ involvement).

Renal tuberculosis may occur as part of a generalized haematogenous dissemination (miliary tuberculosis) in which numerous small discrete 'tubercles' are scattered throughout the kidney parenchyma.

Alternatively there may be massive nodular areas of caseous necrosis involving both cortex and medulla, but centred on the pyramids which undergo necrosis and sloughing (Figures 4.10 and 4.11).

References

1. Heptinstall, R. H. and Gorrill, R. H. (1955). Experimental pyelonephritis and its effect on the blood pressure. *J. Pathol. Bacteriol.*, **69**, 191–198.

2. Heptinstall, R. H. (1974). In *Pathology of the Kidney*, 2nd Edn, p. 878. (Boston: Little, Brown & Co).

3. Rolleston, G. L., Maling, T. M. J. and Hodson, C. J. (1974). Intrarenal reflux and the scarred kidney. *Arch. Dis. Child.*, **49**, 531–539.

4. Hodson, C. J., Maling, T. M. J., McManamon, P. and Lewis, M. G. (1975). The pathogenesis of reflux nephropathy – chronic atrophic pyelonephritis. *Br. J. Radiol.*, Suppl. 13, 1–26.

5. Ransley, P. G. and Risdon, R. A. (1978). Reflux and renal scarring. *Br. J. Radiol.*, **51**, Suppl. 14, 1–35.

6. Kincaid-Smith, P. (1979). Glomerular lesions in atrophic pyelonephritis (PN). In Hodson, C. J. and Kincaid-Smith, P. (eds.) *Reflux Nephropathy* (New York: Masson Publishing).

7. Bhathena, D. B., Weiss, J. H., Holland, N. H., McMorrow, R. G., Curtis, J. J., Lucas, B. A. and Luke, R. G. (1980). Focal and segmental glomerular sclerosis in reflux nephropathy (chronic pyelonephritis). *Am. J. Med.* (in press).

Arteriosclerosis, Benign and Malignant Nephrosclerosis and Renal Artery Stenosis

5

Arteriosclerosis

The most frequent vascular change encountered in the kidneys is some form of arteriosclerosis and this is invariably present to some degree with advancing age. Arteriosclerotic changes vary depending on the size of artery involved:

(i) Atherosclerosis, characterized by the formation of fibro-lipid intimal plaques and identical morphologically to that seen elsewhere in the arterial system, affects the main renal arteries and their larger branches (Figure 5.1). The lesions, and any associated thrombus, may cause renal artery stenosis and lead to hypertension, or may completely occlude an artery and result in renal infarction.

(ii) Intimal fibro-elastic hyperplasia characterized by laminar reduplication of the elastica and an increase in intimal fibrous tissue with consequent luminal narrowing affects muscular arteries of arcuate and interlobular size (Figure 5.2).

(iii) Arteriolosclerosis is the thickening of the walls of small interlobular arteries and afferent arterioles by the deposition of an amorphous eosinophilic hyaline substance beneath the endothelium (Figure 5.3).

The narrowing of the renal arterial vasculature produces a varying degree of ischaemic parenchymal atrophy (Figure 5.4). Patchy tubular atrophy, with tubular narrowing, flattening of the lining epithelium and thickening of the tubular basement membranes, is the most prominent alteration and is usually accompanied by some tubular separation and interstitial fibrosis. Glomerular changes also occur but are generally less extensive, and the majority of glomeruli, even in areas of tubular atrophy, are morphologically normal. The alterations range from shrinkage of the glomerular tufts and thickening of the basement membrane of Bowman's capsule, associated with a minor mesangial increase and a thickening and wrinkling of capillary basement membranes, to more advanced changes with laying down of collagen in the urinary space (Figure 5.5). This collagen deposition starts around the hilum of the tuft and gradually extends to obliterate the urinary space (Figure 5.6). The glomerular tuft gradually loses its cellular component and becomes compressed by the collagenous mantle so that eventually the glomerulus is converted to a rounded, virtually acellular scar. Usually, some of the original tuft structure can still be made out if PAS staining is employed; the collagenous mantle stains poorly whilst the compressed tuft remnant stains magenta. Advanced glomerular sclerosis is most prominent immediately beneath the renal capsule, but the changes are very patchy; completely sclerosed glomeruli occur adjacent to normal ones.

In uncomplicated renal arteriosclerosis, macroscopic changes are confined to a generalized slight thinning of the cortex and a granularity of the subcapsular surface of the kidney reflecting patchy parenchymal atrophy. Sometimes depressed scars due to old infarcts are present. In the absence of hypertension, arteriosclerotic changes are not associated with significant diminution in renal function.

Benign Nephrosclerosis

Essential hypertension is associated with similar changes in the kidney and renal vasculature to those described in renal arteriosclerosis. Arteriolar sclerosis is often particularly prominent. The nature of the hyaline material seen in the arteriolar walls is not completely known, but ultrastructural and immunofluorescent studies suggest that it is derived by deposition of plasma proteins and lipids which leak from the circulation. It is possible that hypertension may injure the endothelium and increase this leakage. Arteriolar sclerosis is particularly severe in diabetic subjects.

In hypertensive patients arteriosclerosis tends to become established at an earlier stage in life than in normotensive people. It is generally accepted that the effect of raised arterial pressure on arterial vessels is to accentuate and accelerate the normal ageing process. The suggestion that the premature arterial changes are a result rather than the cause of hypertension is supported by the observations that some hypertensive patients show no significant vascular abnormalities, whilst many elderly patients with arteriosclerosis are normotensive.

Benign nephrosclerosis alone very rarely causes chronic renal failure, and only 5% of patients with essential hypertension exhibit any renal insufficiency.

Malignant Nephrosclerosis

Rarely malignant (or accelerated) hypertension arises *de novo*; usually, however, it is preceded by a varying period of essential hypertension. Thus, in most cases, changes in the kidney due to malignant hypertension (malignant nephrosclerosis) are superimposed on those of benign nephrosclerosis.

The definitive lesion of accelerated hypertension is 'fibrinoid' arteriolar necrosis (Figure 5.7). The arteriolar walls are necrotic with acellular, brightly eosinophilic material, having the histochemical

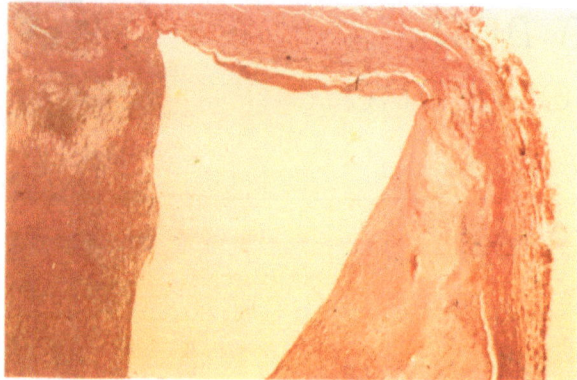

Figure 5.1 Atherosclerosis. Part of the wall of a main renal artery which is partially occluded by a fibro-lipid intimal plaque which is focally calcified. H & E ×144.

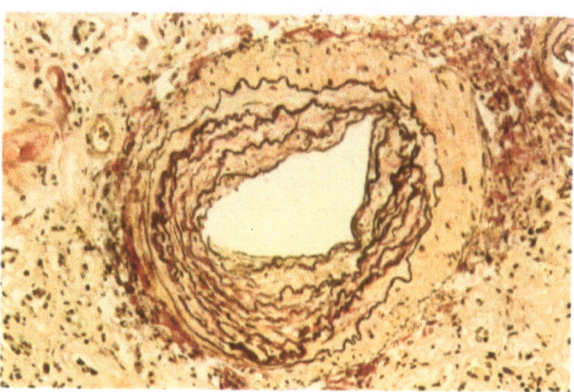

Figure 5.2 Fibro-elastic intimal hyperplasia in an arcuate artery. Elastic–van Gieson ×240.

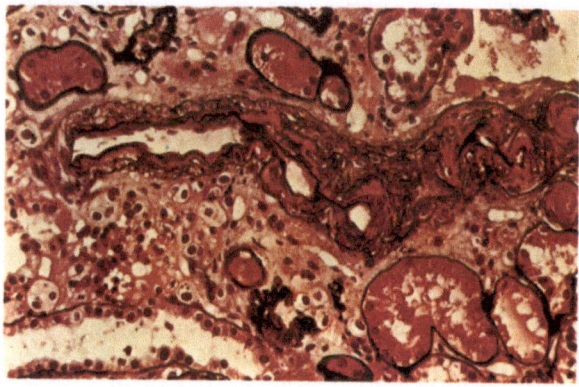

Figure 5.3 Arteriolosclerosis of an afferent arteriole showing hyaline thickening of the wall. H & E ×600.

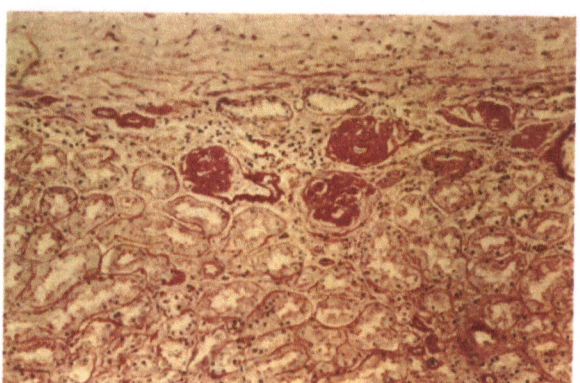

Figure 5.4 Ischaemic glomerular sclerosis affecting glomeruli immediately beneath the renal capsule. There are associated atrophic tubules. PAS ×120.

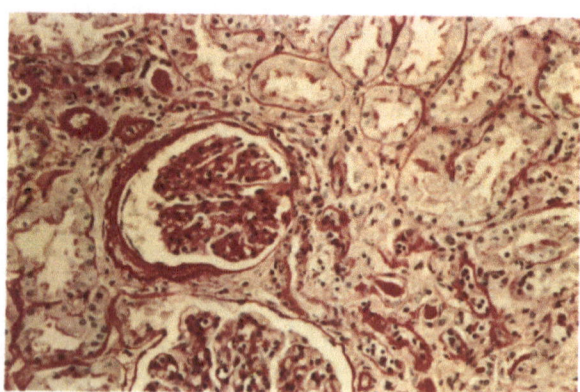

Figure 5.5 Ischaemic glomerular damage showing some shrinkage of the glomerular tuft, collagen deposition on the inside of Bowman's capsule. There is atrophy of the associated tubule. PAS ×360.

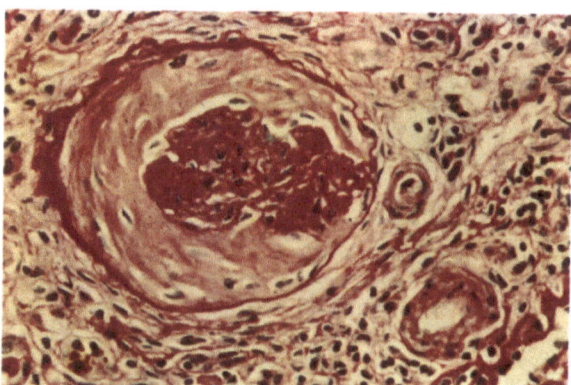

Figure 5.6 Advanced ischaemic glomerular damage. The glomerular tuft is contracted and virtually acellular, and is sharply distinguished from the pale-staining collagen which obliterates the urinary space in this PAS stain section. This differentiation is not well demonstrated by H & E staining. PAS ×480.

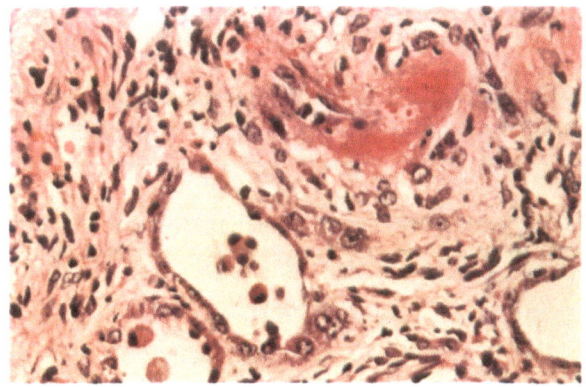

Figure 5.7 Fibrinoid arteriolar necrosis in accelerated hypertension. There is necrosis of the wall of an afferent arteriole with deposition of brightly eosinophilic 'smudgy' material ('fibrinoid'). H & E ×600.

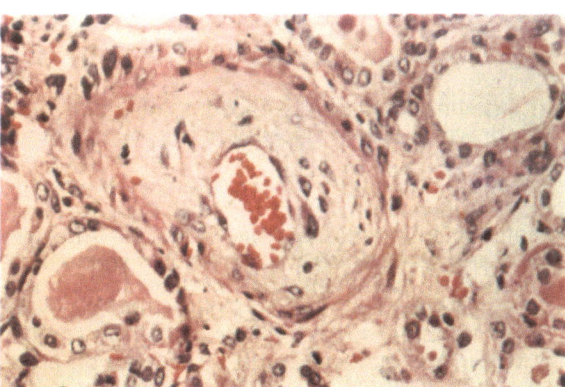

Figure 5.8 Interlobular arterial change in accelerated hypertension. There is marked intimal fibroblastic proliferation, with an increase in ground substance. H & E ×600.

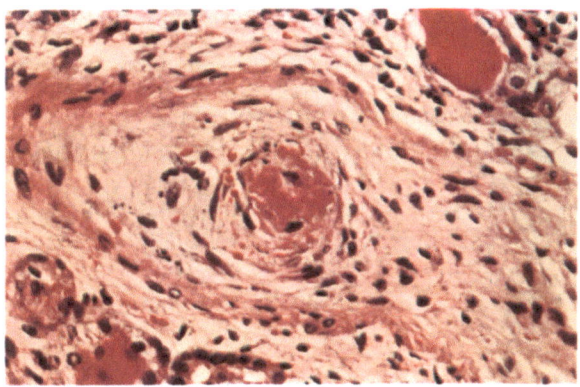

Figure 5.9 Section from the same case as Figure 5.8. The narrowed lumen of this interlobular artery is occluded by a thrombus. H & E ×600.

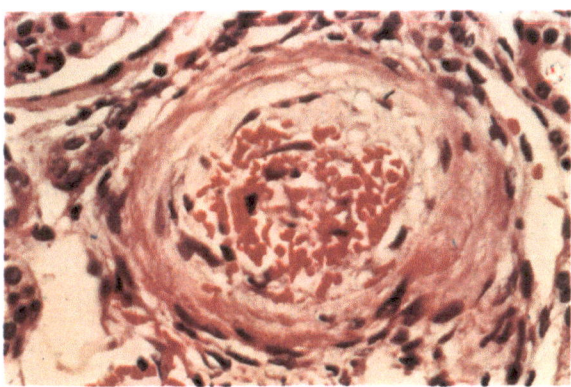

Figure 5.10 Section also from the same case as Figure 5.8, showing extravasation of red blood cells into the thickened intima. H & E ×600.

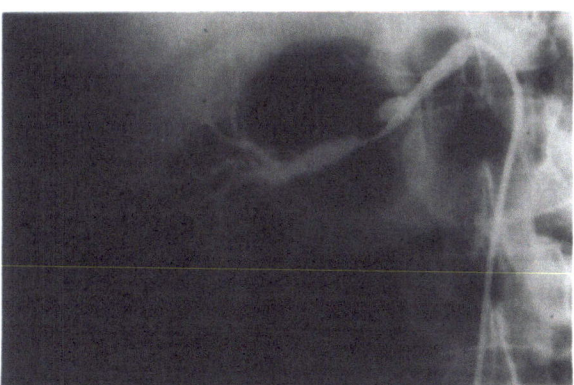

Figure. 5.11 Renal artery stenosis. An angiogram showing a localized narrowing of the right renal artery with post-stenotic dilatation of the vessel distal to it.

and immunofluorescent reactions of fibrin, deposited within them. Occasionally, microthrombi occlude the narrowed arteriolar lumen and sometimes red blood cells permeate the necrotic wall to form microhaemorrhages outside. Inflammatory cells sometimes infiltrate the wall, but although such necrotizing arteriolitis is common in experimental hypertension in animals such as the rat, it is uncommon in human cases. Fibrinoid necrosis of afferent arterioles often extends to involve capillaries within the glomerular tufts. This may be associated with proliferation of cells within the tufts and with capsular crescent formation. Such changes, particularly when present in small biopsy specimens, may be confused with those of glomerulonephritis. Conspicuous changes also occur in interlobular arteries, where concentric proliferation of cells in the intima results in considerable narrowing and often virtual obliteration of their lumina. This is associated with concentric collagen fibre formation, the extent of which appears to be related to the age of the lesion. Often, the thickened intima is basophilic due to an increased amount of ground substance (Figures 5.8, 5.9 and 5.10).

The luminal narrowing of arterial vessels associated with accelerated hypertension causes widespread ischaemic changes, and often scattered areas of infarction in the renal parenchyma. These are usually superimposed on changes of longstanding benign nephrosclerosis.

Macroscopically, there is usually some degree of cortical atrophy, the extent of which depends largely on the duration of pre-existing essential hypertension. In those rare instances where malignant hypertension arises *de novo*, the kidneys may be slightly enlarged with multiple small petechial haemorrhages throughout the cortical tissue.

The factors responsible for precipitating accelerated hypertension are unclear. Fibrinoid arteriolar necrosis appears to be a direct result of the markedly increased arterial pressure, and it has been suggested from experimental observations that overdistension damages the arterioles. This results in seepage of fibrinogen and other plasma proteins into the necrotic arteriolar wall; localized intravascular coagulation may precipitate microthrombus formation in the affected vessels. Increased renin levels are a fairly constant finding in accelerated hypertension and may further increase vascular permeability. Occasionally, a thrombocytopenic haemolytic anaemia accompanies accelerated hypertension. Linton *et al.*[1] have suggested that red cell destruction results from mechanical lysis as the cells traverse the damaged renal microvasculature, and that such lysis would release thromboplastins, adenosine diphosphate and possibly inhibitors of fibrinolysis, thus enhancing fibrin and platelet deposition at the sites of vascular damage. It is further suggested that the 'onion skin' intimal proliferation in the smaller renal arteries is a response to fibrin deposition in these vessels; Kincaid-Smith[2] has emphasized the similarities between the lesions in accelerated hypertension and other thrombotic microangiopathies in which disseminated intravascular coagulation occurs.

Whatever the mechanism precipitating accelerated hypertension, it seems clear that the resulting vascular changes are important in sustaining the high levels of arterial pressure which result. Extensive secondary parenchymal changes develop quickly in untreated patients, and before the introduction of effective hypotensive drugs, patients developed renal failure in the course of only a few months.

Renal Artery Stenosis

Constriction of one main renal artery, or one of its larger branches, may cause hypertension in man. The mechanisms involved are of considerable interest and are reviewed by Wilson *et al.*[3].

Atherosclerosis involving either the renal artery, or more commonly the aorta at the mouth of the renal artery, is the most frequent cause (Figure 5.11). Non-atheromatous fibrous and fibromuscular dysplasias of the renal artery are rarer causes which, unlike atheroma, tend to affect women more often than men and present at an earlier age, usually in the third or fourth decades. McCormack[4] classifies renal artery dysplasias as follows:

(1) Intimal dysplasia – characterized by intimal thickening inside the internal elastic lamina.

(2) Medial fibroplasia with aneurysm formation. Fibrosis here is more medial than intimal and is patchy. The intervening areas show thinning of the media with aneurysm formation producing a characteristic 'string of beads' appearance on arteriography.

(3) Subadventitial fibroplasia – a cuff of fibrosis replaces the outer media.

(4) Fibromuscular hyperplasia in which a haphazard arrangement of muscle and collagen bundles is seen in the media.

Unusual causes of renal artery stenosis include aortitis (Takayashu's disease), thrombosis or aneurysm formation in the renal artery and extrinsic pressure by tumours, enlarged lymph nodes or abnormal fibromuscular bands.

The kidney supplied by the stenotic renal artery is usually reduced in size with evidence of diffuse ischaemic atrophy and widespread tubular atrophy, glomerular crowding and sclerosis, interstitial fibrosis and focal inflammatory cell infiltration. Sometimes fresh or old infarcts are present. Because the diminished renal perfusion is a stimulus to renin secretion, hyperplasia of the juxtamedullary apparatus may be apparent. Since the stenotic renal artery protects vessels in the ischaemic kidney from the effects of hypertension, arteriosclerosis is no more marked than would be expected for the patient's age. However, the contralateral unprotected kidney may show changes of benign or malignant nephrosclerosis depending on the duration and severity of the hypertension.

References

1. Linton, A. L., Gavras, H., Gleadle, R. I., Hutchinson, H. E., Lawson, D. H., Lever, A. F., MacAdam, R. F., McNicol, G. P. and Robertson, J. I. S. (1969). Microangiopathic haemolytic anaemia and the pathogenesis of malignant hypertension. *Lancet*, **1**, 1277–1282.

2. Kincaid-Smith, P. (1975). Participation of intravascular coagulation in the pathogenesis of glomerular and vascular lesions. *Kidney Int.*, **7**, 242–253.

3. Wilson, C., Ledingham, J. M. and Floyer, M. A. (1971). Experimental renal and renoprival hypertension. In Rouiller, C. and Muller, A. F. (eds.) *The Kidney*. (New York: Academic Press).

4. McCormack, L. J. (1973). Morphological abnormalities of the renal artery associated with hypertension. In Onesti, G. and Kim, K. E. (eds.) *High Blood Pressure*. (New York: Grune and Stratton).

Renal Infarction, Cortical Necrosis and Tubular Necrosis

6

Renal Infarction

Ischaemic necrosis of the kidney (renal infarction) usually results from arterial obstruction; its extent depends largely on the size and number of vessels involved. Arterial occlusion is most frequently due to thrombo-embolism by thrombus formed within the heart cavities as a complication of myocardial infarction, atrial fibrillation or infective endocarditis. Occlusion may also be due to local causes within the renal arterial system such as atherosclerosis or thrombosis associated with periarteritis.

The changes in the kidney following arterial occlusion have been followed experimentally in animals and available evidence suggests a similar sequence in man. An early infarct is dark red and sharply demarcated, forming a cone-shaped zone with its base at the capsule surface and its apex at the cortico-medullary junction. Microscopically there is profound congestion of glomerular and intertubular capillaries.

The next stage is the development of coagulative necrosis in which the nuclei disappear from the infarcted area, leaving the basic pattern of cellular architecture intact (Figure 6.1). This process starts peripherally and progresses towards the centre of the lesion. Gradually, during the course of a few days, the infarct becomes paler, and its cut surface changes from grey to yellow, as gradual breakdown of red blood cells occurs (Figure 6.2). This process begins at the centre of the infarct and spreads outwards, the haemorrhagic rim gradually disappearing after about a week. Neutrophil polymorphs infiltrate the peripheral zone of the infarct and beneath the renal capsule. These polymorphs undergo karyorrhexis during the first few days and after one week are seen only as 'nuclear dust' (Figures 6.3 and 6.4). Reparative fibrosis occurs at the margins of an infarct whilst its centre gradually collapses and shrinks. The capsular surface of the infarct becomes indented and gradually forms a depressed scar in the renal surface; occasionally calcification occurs in the central necrotic zone.

In the marginal zone between the infarct and surrounding healthy parenchyma some necrosis and regeneration of proximal convoluted tubules occurs. Areas of tubular loss with persistence of glomeruli are frequently seen around infarcts. Occasionally, segmented necrosis and epithelial hyperplasia of glomeruli occurs in this marginal zone. Epithelial proliferation may be sufficiently marked to produce 'capsular crescents'. Scarring following segmented tuft necrosis may result in capsular adhesions. Both these features may cause confusion with glomerulonephritis, particularly when seen in needle biopsy specimens. Clinically renal infarcts are usually silent although large infarcts may cause loin pain and haematuria. Occasionally transient hypertension occurs.

Venous infarction of the kidney is comparatively rare and is an occasional complication of renal vein thrombosis. It is most frequently seen in dehydrated infants or as a complication of intra-abdominal sepsis (Figures 6.5 and 6.6). The infarction produced is intensely haemorrhagic and in infants the whole kidney is usually involved.

Renal Cortical Necrosis

Traditionally, this term is applied to bilateral, confluent, ischaemic necrosis involving almost all the renal cortex (except for the subcapsular and deep juxtamedullary zones) and sparing the medulla (Figure 6.7). This gross form is almost invariably fatal, although fortunately rare. It is now recognized, however, that much less extensive focal and patchy forms of renal cortical necrosis occur which are probably much more common than the gross form, and are compatible with recovery. Usually the condition is associated with complications of pregnancy such as premature placental separation, placenta praevia, severe toxaemia or septic abortion. It may, however, accompany any cause of severe peripheral circulatory failure, for example, extensive burns, gastro-intestinal haemorrhage, bacteraemia or septicaemia.

Histologically, there is coagulative, ischaemic necrosis of glomeruli and tubules. Glomerular necrosis may be associated with fibrin thrombi in the glomerular tufts and occasionally in afferent arterioles. In the minor, focal forms only a few glomeruli are necrotic in any given area, and not infrequently some ischaemic foci exhibit only tubular necrosis (Figure 6.8). With more extensive cortical necrosis, the walls of larger blood vessels are also necrotic and often occluded by thrombi.

The pathogenesis of renal cortical necrosis is unclear. Sheehan and Moore[1] regarded intense prolonged spasm of muscular arteries within the kidney as the primary factor leading to cortical ischaemia and subsequent necrosis. Following relaxation of vasospasm, blood flow into the necrotic arteries and smaller vessels results in thrombosis. Other investigations, notably McKay[2], consider generalized intravascular coagulation, with blockage of small vessels including those of the renal cortex, to be the principal cause of renal cortical necrosis. In experimental animals the generalized Swartzman reaction, elicited by two small doses of bacterial endotoxin given 24 hours apart, results in disseminated intravascular coagulation (DIC) and renal cortical necrosis. A similar reaction occurs in preg-

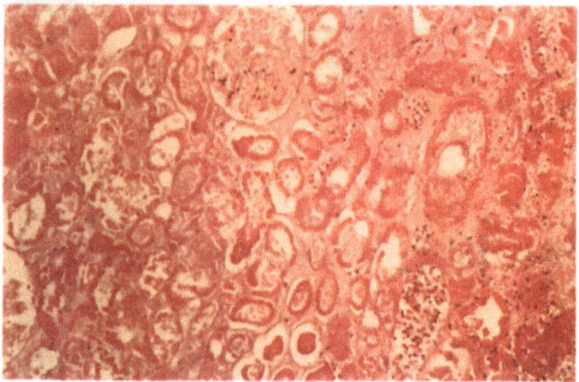

Figure 6.1 Coagulative necrosis at the centre of a renal infarct. Nuclear detail is virtually lost, but the 'ghosts' of glomeruli, tubules and vessels are still clearly visible. H & E   × 240.

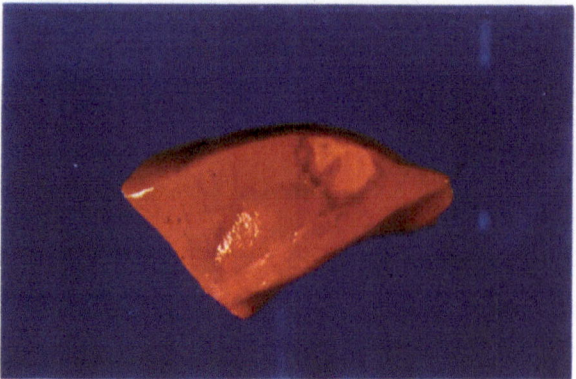

Figure 6.2 Wedge-shaped area of cortical infarction. The centre is pale and yellow indicating that it is at least a few days old. This is surrounded by a haemorrhagic rim.

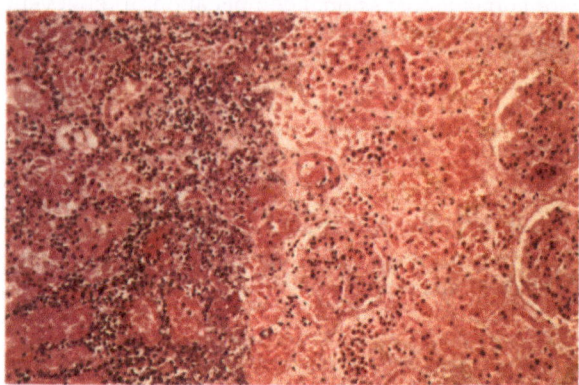

Figure 6.3 Zone of neutrophil infiltration at the edge of an infarct. Many of the polymorphs have undergone karyorrhexis and appear as nuclear dust. H & E   × 240.

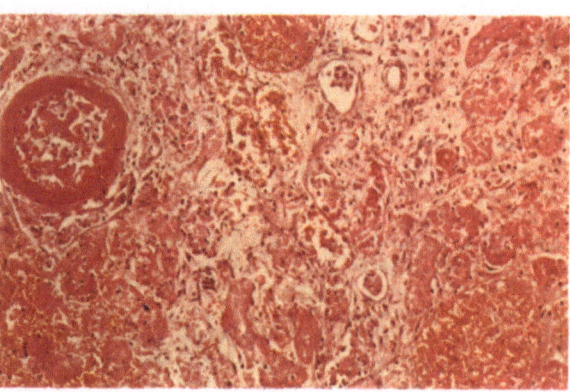

Figure 6.4 Renal cortical infarct in which a necrotic interlobular artery is occluded by fibrin. H & E   × 240.

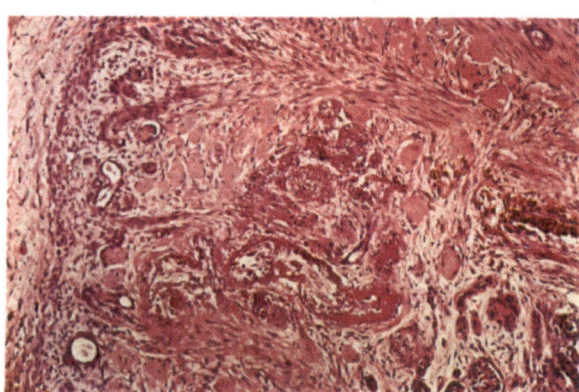

Figure 6.5 Venous infarction in a baby dying at 9 weeks. At the age of 1 week, presented with severe dehydration and renal vein thrombosis. The cortex is necrotic with areas of fibroblastic proliferation and mainly tubular calcification. H & E   × 60.

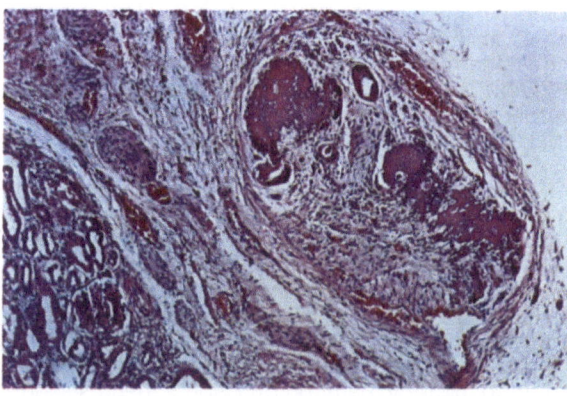

Figure 6.6 From the same patient as Figure 6.5 showing organized and partially calcified thrombus within a large renal vein. H & E   × 60.

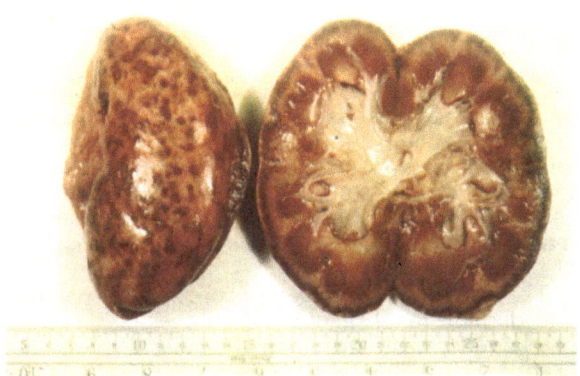

Figure 6.7 The kidneys from a patient dying of bilateral renal cortical necrosis. The whole of the cortex is pale apart from blotchy haemorrhagic zones beneath the capsular surface.

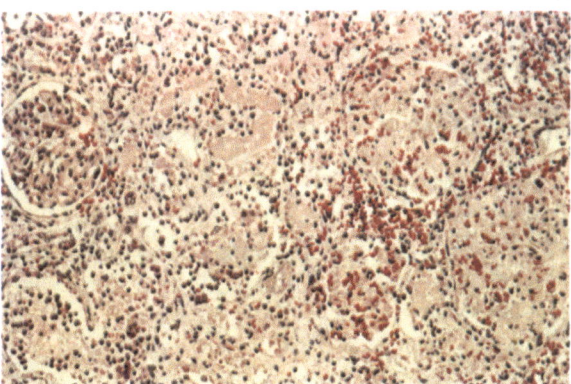

Figure 6.8 Focal renal cortical necrosis showing coagulative necrosis of tubules and two glomeruli. A third glomerulus is unaffected. H & E × 240.

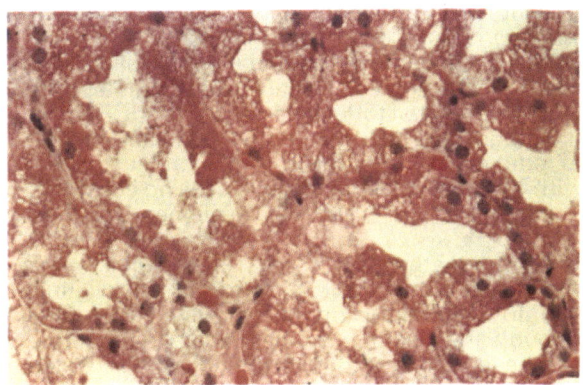

Figure 6.9 Conspicuous cytoplasmic vacuolation of tubular epithelial cells. This change may represent an early and probably recoverable stage of tubular necrosis; and may be seen both in ischaemic and nephrotoxic lesions. H & E × 480.

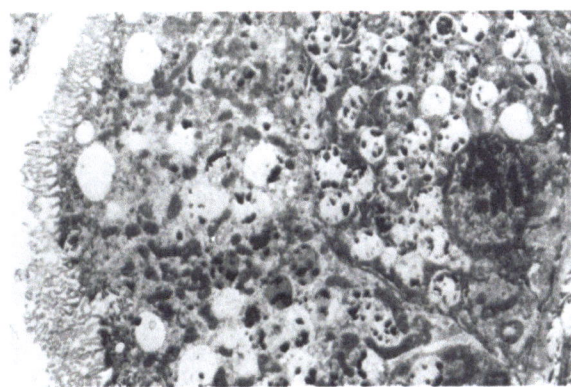

Figure 6.10 Electron micrograph from the same case as Figure 6.9. The vacuoles are membrane-bound and contain conspicuous electron dense deposits near the inner aspect of the membranes. × 4500.

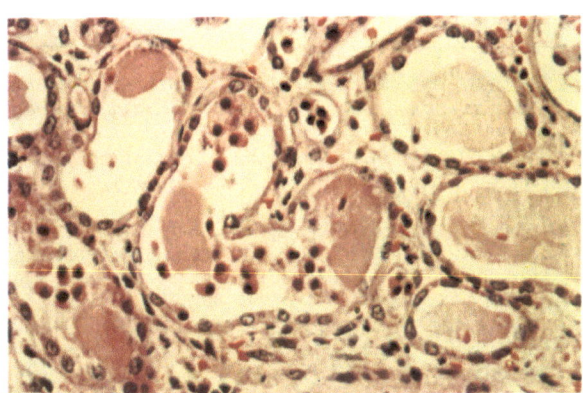

Figure 6.11 Fully-developed acute tubular necrosis. The majority of tubular cells are necrotic and many are desquamating into the tubular lumina. H & E × 480.

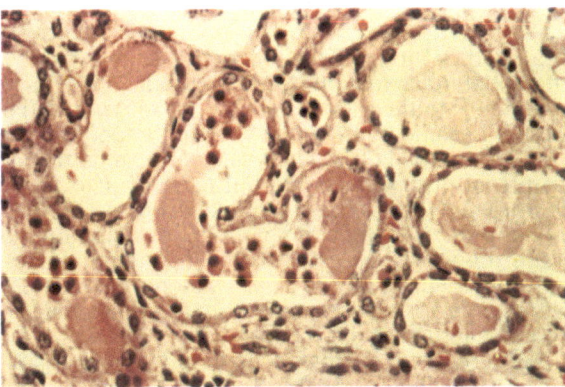

Figure 6.12 From the same case as Figure 6.11. The tubules are dilated and lined by a low, regenerative epithelium. Some tubules contain desquamated necrotic cells within their lumen. It should be emphasized that tubular necrosis and evidence of tubular regeneration frequently co-exist. H & E × 480.

nant animals with a single dose of endotoxin. Clinical evidence of DIC may be found in conditions such as bacteraemic shock and obstetric emergencies which may be associated with renal cortical necrosis. However, DIC and fibrin deposition within glomerular capillaries may occur in the absence of renal cortical necrosis so that the development of this lesion probably also requires a degree of vascular spasm.

Acute Tubular Necrosis

This may be due to:

(i) Direct poisoning of the tubular epithelium mainly affecting proximal convoluted tubules (the nephrotoxic lesion), or

(ii) Acute ischaemic damage affecting all parts of the renal tubules (the tubulorrhexic lesion), or to a combination of (i) and (ii).

Nephrotoxic tubular necrosis can be produced by a variety of poisons (see Table 6.1). Histologically there is necrosis of proximal tubular epithelial cells,

Table 6.1   Some nephrotoxins associated with acute tubular necrosis

Metals and ions	Antibiotics and other drugs
Mercury	Sulphonamides
Gold	Methicillin
Lead	Neomycin
Arsenic	Polymyxin
Bismuth	Gentamycin
Chromium	Amphotericin B
Uranium	Kanamycin
Phosphorus	Cephalothin
	Cephaloridine
	Methoxyflurane
Organic compounds	Mephenesin
Glycols (ethylene and diethylene)	Quinine
Carbon tetrachloride	Other
Chloroform	Pesticides
Toluene	Poisonous mushrooms
Phenol	Contrast media

tubular dilatation, interstitial oedema and patchy interstitial inflammation. Necrotic tubular cells desquamate into the tubular lumina but in general the tubular basement membranes remain intact. Swelling and vacuolation of epithelial cells is a particular feature of glycol poisoning but can occur to some degree in any form of acute tubular necrosis (Figures 6.9 and 6.10). Depending when examination is made there may be evidence of regeneration. Regenerative epithelial cells are flattened or cuboidal with large, irregular nuclei; occasional mitotic figures can usually be recognized.

Tubulorrhexic necrosis follows prolonged hypotension leading to renal ischaemia. Common precipitating causes include crushing injuries and burns, obstetric catastrophies such as accidental haemorrhage, severe dehydration, peritonitis and acute haemolysis. It is evident that many of these conditions may also be associated with renal cortical necrosis, although the degree of renal ischaemia required to cause cortical necrosis is generally

greater and more prolonged. Microscopically tubulorrhexic necrosis is characterized by variable degrees of patchy tubular necrosis (Figures 6.11 and 6.12) involving not only the proximal but also the distal tubules and loops of Henle[3]. This is associated with disruption of the tubular basement membranes. Pigment containing tubular casts are also a frequent finding.

The relationship between acute tubular necrosis and oliguric renal failure is controversial[4]. Tubular blockage by casts or necrotic cellular debris is unlikely to contribute significantly to oliguria, since this usually occurs early in the process, whilst casts take several days to develop, and in any case their number correlates poorly with the degree of renal failure.

It has been proposed that oliguria is due to a profound fall in glomerular filtration rate, and that tubular necrosis is merely a secondary ischaemic effect having no primary role in acute renal failure. It is true that in some patients with hypotension due to peripheral circulatory failure, marked diminution in urine output occurs in the absence of readily recognizable damage to tubular epithelial cells, and that often the degree of renal failure correlates poorly with the extent of tubular necrosis when it is present. It is suggested that marked hypotension may lead to renin release from the juxtaglomerular apparatus, with formation of angiotensin II causing constriction of afferent arterioles and a fall in glomerular filtration rate.

An alternative hypothesis, affording a primary role to the tubular lesions, suggests that oliguria is due to back diffusion of the glomerular filtrate through the necrotic epithelial cells. This process has been elegantly demonstrated in rats rendered anuric with mercuric chloride using the dye lissamine green[5], and continued glomerular filtration in the presence of acute renal failure has been shown radiologically[6, 7].

It is probable that both these mechanisms may be important to differing degrees and at different stages in the clinical course of the disease.

References

1. Sheehan, H. L. and Moore, H. C. (1952). *Renal Cortical Necrosis and the Kidney of Concealed Accidental Haemorrhage*. (Oxford: Blackwell).

2. McKay, D. G. (1965). *Disseminated Intravascular Coagulation: An Intermediary Mechanism of Disease*, p. 431. (New York: Harper and Row).

3. Oliver, J., MacDowell, M. and Tracy A. (1951). The pathogenesis of acute renal failure associated with traumatic and toxic injury: Renal ischaemia, nephrotoxic damage and the ischaemic episode. *J. Clin. Invest.*, **30**, 1307–1440.

4. Dunnill, M. S. and Jerrome, D. W. (1976). Renal tubular necrosis due to shock: light- and electron-microscope observations. *J. Pathol.*, **118**, 109–112.

5. Bank, N., Mutz, B. F. and Aynedjian, H. S. (1967). The role of 'leakage' of tubular fluid in anuria due to mercury poisoning. *J. Clin. Invest.*, **46**, 695–704.

6. Fry, I. K. and Cattell, W. R. (1970). The IVP in renal failure. *Br. J. Hosp. Med.*, **3**, 67–71.

7. Chamberlain, M. J. and Sherwood, T. (1967). Intravenous urography in experimental acute renal failure in the rat. *Nephron*, **4**, 65–74.

Although primary glomerular diseases such as glomerulonephritis frequently have associated secondary interstitial lesions, it is necessary to distinguish them from cases where there is no primary glomerular damage and the pathological changes affect predominantly the tubules and interstitium. For this purpose, the description 'interstitial nephritis' is used, and although it includes a variety of different diseases of known and unknown aetiology, the breadth of the term has some merits. A label of 'interstitial nephritis' prompts careful evaluation of all the relevant clinical and pathological aspects before a more precise diagnosis is attempted. Microscopically, interstitial nephritides are principally characterized by changes in the interstitium (oedema and/or fibrosis, often with inflammatory cell infiltration) and the tubules (tubular atrophy and loss). These lesions may result from direct damage to tubules or interstitium, or from vascular insufficiency. Sometimes a combination of factors is involved and frequently the exact mechanisms are obscure. Although glomerular damage is not a primary feature of interstitial nephritis, secondary (usually 'ischaemic') lesions may develop in some glomeruli.

The principal causes of interstitial nephritis are listed in Table 7.1.

Table 7.1   Interstitial nephritis

Pyelonephritis (reflux nephropathy)   (see Chapter 4)
Renal vascular disease
Benign and malignant nephrosclerosis ⎫
Arteriosclerosis   ⎬ (see Chapter 5)
Renal artery stenosis   ⎭
Some types of allograph rejection   (see Chapter 16)
Obstructive uropathy
Drugs (e.g. methicillin, analgesic nephropathy)
Irradiation
Heavy metal poisoning (e.g. cadmium, lead)
Metabolic disorders (e.g. gout, nephrocalcinosis, cystinosis)
Nephronophthisis   (see Chapter 3)
Balkan nephropathy

Obstructive Uropathy

Obstruction at any level in the urinary tract from the renal pelvis to the urethra leads to dilatation of the renal pelvis and calyces (hydronephrosis). Depending on the degree and duration of the obstruction, a varying amount of atrophy of the renal parenchyma occurs (Figure 7.1). In longstanding obstruction, the whole kidney may be markedly enlarged and the parenchyma reduced to a thin shell overlying the greatly dilated pelvi-calyceal system (Figure 7.2).

Microscopical changes are at first most prominent in the medulla. Dilatation of the calyces leads to flattening and atrophy of the pyramids whose tubules appear tangentially rather than radially aligned and are often dilated. There is an accompanying increase in interstitial fibrous tissue. Initially, changes in the cortex may not be obvious apart from the gradual decrease in thickness. Later there is widespread tubular atrophy and loss with diffuse interstitial fibrosis; glomeruli are well preserved until a late stage when global sclerosis occurs. Patchy interstitial fibrosis and chronic inflammation is also present. Arteriosclerotic changes are variable and are usually most marked in cases with hypertension. Urinary obstruction is often accompanied by pyelonephritis but microscopically changes due to infection may be difficult to distinguish from those due to obstruction. Inflammatory changes in the renal pelvis are associated with the presence of infection in the upper renal tract. Macroscopic examination of the subcapsular surface of the kidney may also be helpful; segmental scarring usually indicates infection and in uncomplicated hydronephrosis the renal surface is often surprisingly smooth. Sudden complete obstruction, which may occur, for example, with impaction of a renal calculus or accidential surgical ligation of the ureter is often associated with diffuse renal atrophy rather than dilatation. Sometimes, however, hydronephrotic dilatation of the kidney occurs even with complete obstruction. This implies continued urine production, and it is postulated that urine drainage may continue by pyelovenous or possible pyelolymphatic reabsorption.

Drug Reactions

(i) Acute Interstitial Nephritis

Hypersensitivity to certain drugs, especially penicillin derivatives, may produce a form of interstitial nephritis. Although first described with sulphonamides, this reaction most commonly occurs with methicillin. Other drugs which have been implicated include ampicillin, penicillin, cephalothin and phenindione[1].

Clinically, proteinuria, haematuria and a rising serum creatinine are accompanied by fever, skin rashes and eosinophilia. Acute renal failure may develop. Symptoms usually begin abruptly, some two weeks after drug treatment is started. This sudden onset accounts for the description of the renal lesion as acute interstitial nephritis, although the tissue inflammatory reaction is largely chronic in type (Figure 7.3). The histological changes in the kidney at onset are widespread interstitial oedema

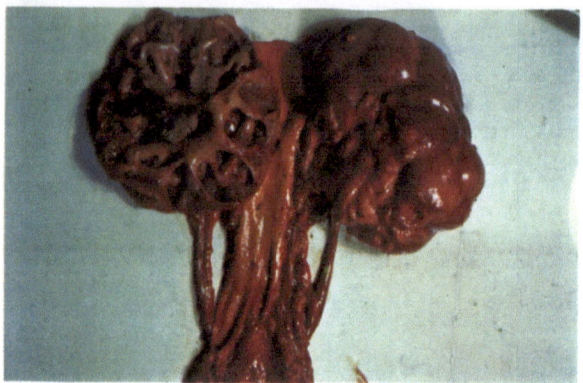

Figure 7.1   Obstructive uropathy. Bilateral hydronephrosis in an elderly male with prostatic hypertrophy.

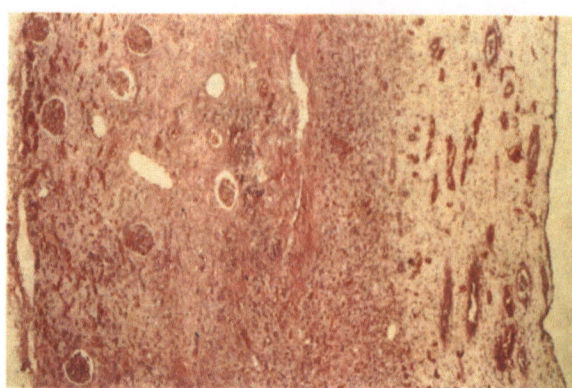

Figure 7.2   Obstructive uropathy. The section shows the full thickness of the parenchyma. There is medullary atrophy, with widespread cortical tubular loss, and interstitial fibrosis. H & E   × 60.

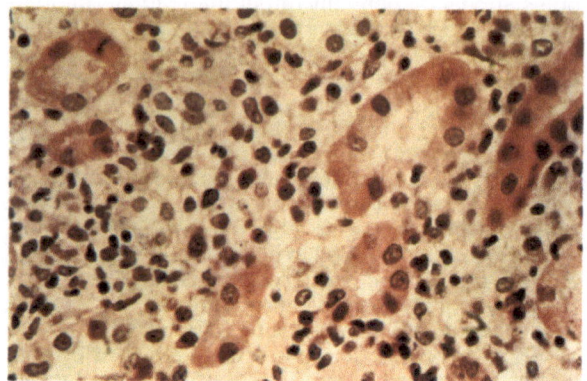

Figure 7.3   Acute interstitial nephritis. Active tubular damage with interstitial oedema and a mixed active chronic inflammatory cell infiltrate. H & E   × 720.

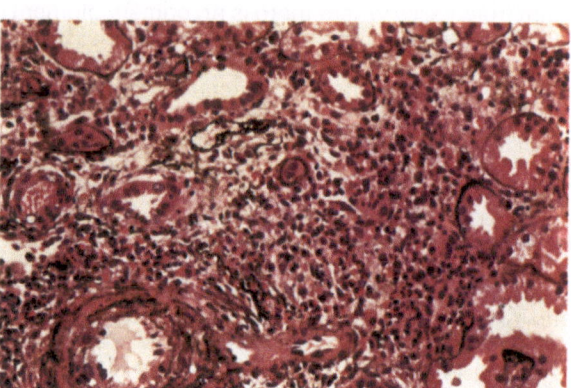

Figure 7.4   Acute interstitial nephritis. Active chronic interstitial inflammation with prominent eosinophils. Biopsy from a patient treated with methicillin. Methenamine Silver/H & E   × 360.

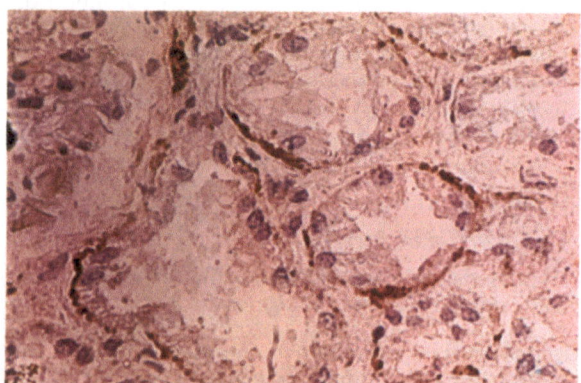

Figure 7.5   Acute interstitial nephritis. Immunoperoxidase staining to show linear deposition of immunoglobulin (IgG) along tubular basement membrane.   × 720.

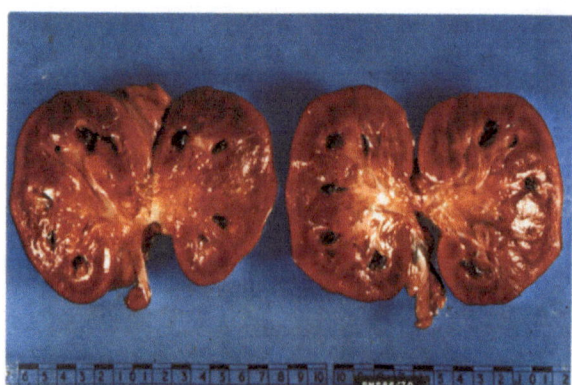

Figure 7.6   Analgesic nephropathy. Bilateral papillary necrosis: the necrotic papillae are blackened. The kidneys from a 51-year-old man who had taken large doses of Codeine co. for many years.

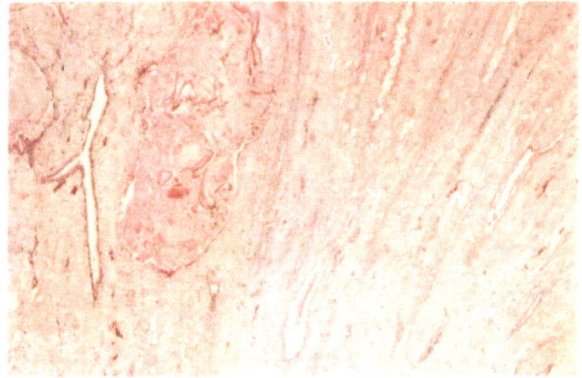

Figure 7.7 Analgesic nephropathy. Necrotic renal papilla with occasional surviving papillary ducts. The majority of papillary ducts appear as 'ghost' structures. H & E ×120.

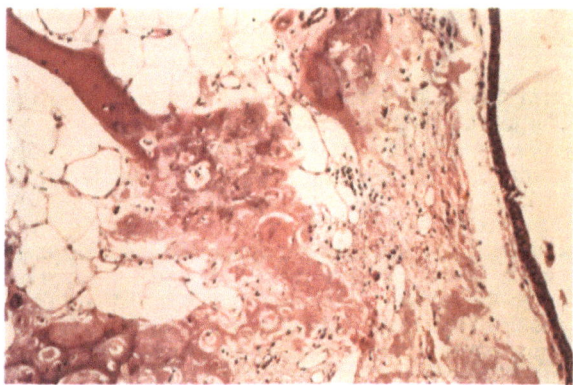

Figure 7.8 Analgesic nephropathy. Calcification and osseous metaplasia in a necrotic papilla. H & E ×120.

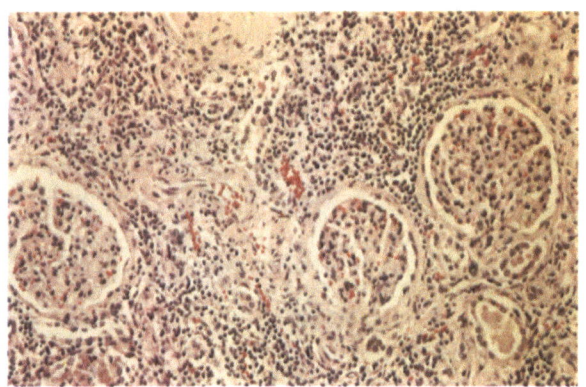

Figure 7.9 Analgesic nephropathy. Chronic interstitial nephritis in the cortex overlying a necrotic papilla. There is conspicuous tubular atrophy and loss with interstitial chronic inflammatory cell infiltration and fibrosis. H & E ×240.

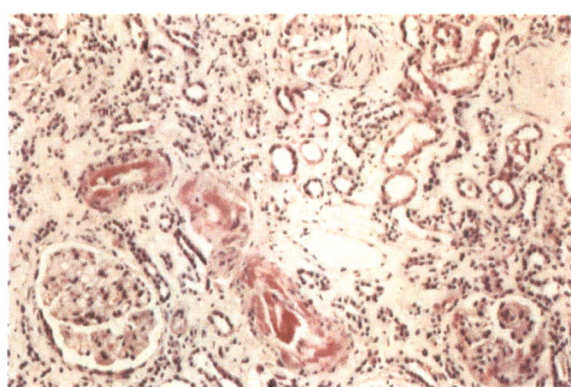

Figure 7.10 Radiation nephritis. Section of a biopsy from a 32-year-old man who developed proteinuria and hypertension two years after receiving abdominal radiotherapy for Hodgkin's disease. There is widespread tubular atrophy and an interlobular artery shows prominent 'fibrinoid' necrosis of its wall. H & E ×240.

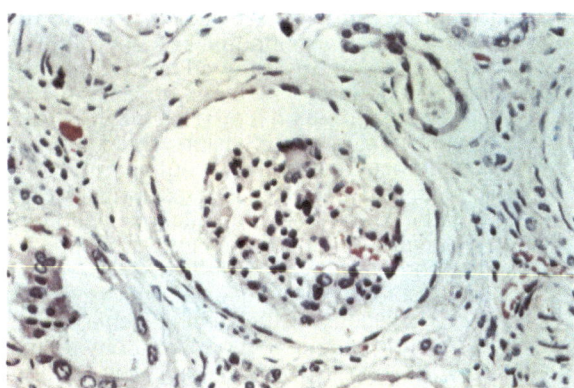

Figure 7.11 Cystinosis. A glomerulus from a three-month-old child showing a characteristic multinucleate epithelial cell in the glomerular tuft. H & E ×480.

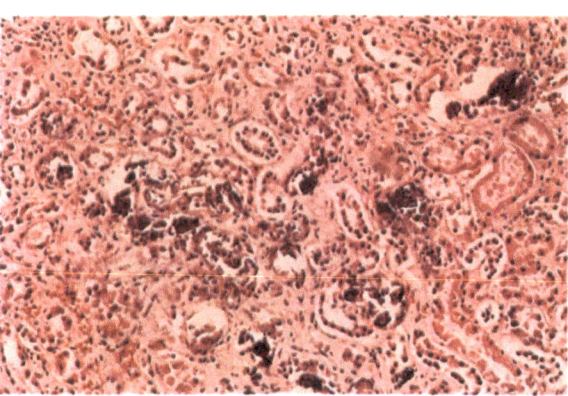

Figure 7.12 Nephrocalcinosis. Tubular and interstitial calcareous deposits in a patient with hypercalcaemia due to widespread metastatic carcinoma in bone. H & E ×120.

and a mixed inflammatory cell infiltrate composed of lymphocytes, histiocytes, plasma cells and occasional neutrophils and eosinophils (Figure 7.4). Tubular changes are prominent though patchy, with foci of necrosis, regeneration and atrophy; the glomeruli are normal. Withdrawal of the offending drug is usually followed by recovery but occasionally chronic renal disease develops and is accompanied by diffuse interstitial fibrosis. The pathogenesis of this type of interstitial nephritis is obscure. Immunofluorescence microscopy in a case associated with methicillin therapy[2] demonstrated linear deposits of IgG and the penicilloyl haptenic group of methicillin along the tubular basement membranes (TBMs). Anti-TBM antibodies were also demonstrated in the serum. It was proposed that conjugates of the penicilloyl hapten with TBM stimulated the formation of anti-TBM antibodies and that these were responsible for the tubular and interstitial damage seen (see also Figure 7.5).

(ii) Nephropathy of Analgesic Abuse

Longterm intensive ingestion of analgesics may occur in chronic painful illnesses like rheumatoid arthritis or as a form of drug abuse, and can result in chronic renal disease. The pathological changes in the kidneys affect both cortex and medulla. Some or all of the renal papillae undergo necrosis (Figure 7.6). Histologically, the necrotic papillae are structureless, virtually acellular and eosinophilic. Often the outlines of the papillary tubules are still recognizable (Figure 7.7), and can be more clearly defined in reticulin preparations. The upper margin of the necrotic papilla is indistinct and merges imperceptibly with the proximal part of the pyramid. Calcification and even osseous metaplasia are common in the necrotic zone (Figure 7.8). A chronic interstitial nephritis develops in the cortex overlying necrotic papillae with widespread diffuse interstitial fibrosis, tubular atrophy and loss, and patchy interstitial inflammation (Figure 7.9). In contrast the glomeruli are usually well preserved, but some focal obsolescence, 'ischaemic' change and periglomerular fibrosis is often seen. The cortical changes are regarded as secondary to the papillary necrosis since their distribution is segmental, directly overlying the necrotic papillae, whilst the columns of Bertin are spared. Furthermore, the papillary necrosis can be shown to precede the development of the cortical lesions[3].

The pathogenesis of analgesic nephropathy is obscure. Phenacetin is the drug most commonly implicated but this is difficult to confirm since it is nearly always dispensed as a mixture with other drugs, such as aspirin and caffeine[4]. Occasional cases are described where aspirin alone appears to be responsible. It is possible that analgesic mixtures have an additive or synergistic effect. The principal pathogenic mechanisms proposed in the development of papillary necrosis are an interference with the medullary blood supply, or a direct 'toxic' action; possibly following concentration of the drug in the medulla[5, 6].

Radiation Nephritis

Radiation damage to the kidneys may occur inadvertently during X-ray therapy of malignant tumours. Clinically it is characterized by impaired renal function, proteinuria and often hypertension.

A variable interval of a few months to several years may occur between irradiation and the onset of clinical symptoms. Affected kidneys may be of normal size or diffusely contracted. The renal capsule is thickened and may be fused with sclerotic tissue in the retroperitoneum around the kidney. The pelvicalyceal system and ureter are normal. Microscopically, tubular atrophy and interstitial fibrosis are present in a patchy or diffuse distribution depending on the severity of the changes. Many glomeruli are normal, but some show fusion of capillary loops, thickening of capillary walls or more advanced hyalinization. Arteries of arcuate and segmental size show patchy intimal thickening. Large interlobular arteries show fine collagenous or cellular intimal thickening. Fibrinoid necrosis is often present in the smaller interlobular arteries and arterioles (Figure 7.10).

Experimental evidence suggests that much of the parenchymal change is a direct result of irradiation rather than a secondary ischaemic affect of the vascular lesions, and this is borne out by the fact that in human cases advanced interstitial nephritis occasionally occurs in the absence of marked vascular changes.

Fibrinoid necrosis of small vessels appears to result from a combination of irradiation effects and hypertension. It has been suggested that irradiation damage to the vessel wall weakens it, so rendering it more prone to fibrinoid necrosis as the arterial pressure rises. Certainly fibrinoid necrosis often occurs with only modest degrees of hypertension following irradiation.

Balkan Nephropathy

This is a remarkable form of chronic interstitial nephritis, the incidence of which is confined to certain localized areas of Yugoslavia, Rumania and Bulgaria, close to the Danube and its tributaries. These are rural areas with a high rainfall. It is suggested that more than 20 000 people may be affected. Clinically, patients develop slowly progressive renal failure with proteinuria and often microscopic haematuria. The usual symptoms are weakness, malaise, a dull loin pain and often a peculiar coppery-grey skin discoloration. Pathologically the kidneys are of equal size and diffusely contracted with thinning of the cortex and blurring of the cortico-medullary junctions. Papillary necrosis is a rare event and when it does occur it does not appear to be the primary lesion since cortical scarring is diffuse rather than confined to areas overlying necrotic papillae. Microscopically, the changes in the kidney are an interstitial nephritis with widespread tubular atrophy, interstitial fibrosis and patchy chronic interstitial inflammation. Some glomerular obsolescence is usually present and is most marked adjacent to the renal capsule. Blood vessels show little change beyond a patchy intimal thickening of larger arteries. About one-third of cases of Balkan nephropathy are complicated by the development of transitional cell tumours at multiple sites in the urinary tract. Similar tumours occasionally complicate analgesic nephropathy although their incidence is much less.

The pathogenesis of Balkan nephropathy is unknown. Residence in endemic areas for at least fifteen years is usual before the diagnosis is made and there is no evidence of a genetic cause. Recently, in the search for local environmental factors, interest has focused on the possible aetiological role of fungi which are frequent contaminants of food stuffs in the damp endemic areas. In particular, heavy fungal contamination of local food stuffs by *Penicillium verrucosum* var. *cyclopium* has been noted. Recent experimental studies have shown consistent renal tubular lesions in rats force-fed cultures of this fungus obtained from maize stored in an endemic area[7].

Metabolic Defects

Interstitial nephritis, usually with a patchy distribution, may be a feature of some metabolic disorders, such as gout, nephrocalcinosis and cystinosis.

The renal lesion in gout is characterized by areas of interstitial fibrosis and tubular atrophy. Urate crystals may be identified within tubules and in the interstitium as birefringent basophilic structures with an amorphous or spindle shape. Collections of elongated crystals may be arranged like the spokes of a wheel and are often surrounded by multinucleate foreign body giant cells. Although best preserved in alcohol-fixed tissues, they can also be identified in formalin-fixed material. Arteriosclerosis is often prominent, and 'ischaemic' changes affect some glomeruli. It is recognized that there is an increased incidence of hypertension in patients with gout.

Nephrocalcinosis is characterized by deposits of calcium salts both in tubular epithelial cells and in the interstitium (Figure 7.12) and may occur both with elevated and depressed levels of serum calcium. Patchy interstitial fibrosis and tubular atrophy may occur and, when severe, nephrocalcinosis may be recognized on plain radiographs of the abdomen.

Nephropathic cystinosis is a recessively inherited disease presenting during the first year of life and characterized by the deposition of L-cystine in many organs including the kidney. The clinical effects are related to functional renal tubular defects and include polyuria, failure to thrive, renal rickets, aminoaciduria, glycosuria, acidosis and hypokalaemia. Morphological changes in the kidney include widespread tubular atrophy, interstitial fibrosis and patchy glomerular hyalinization.

Cystine crystals are deposited in the interstitium and epithelial cells in the glomerular tufts may undergo giant cell transformation (polykaryocytes) (Figure 7.11). Spear[8] has described glomerular epithelial cells and cells in the renal interstitium in which the cytoplasm appears dark in plastic embedded material, possibly representing a reaction product formed by the interaction of cystine with osmium tetroxide.

References

1. Heptinstall, R. H. (1976). Interstitial nephritis. A brief review. *Am. J. Pathol.*, **83**, 214–236.

2. Border, W. A., Lehman, D. H., Egan, J. D., Sass, H. J., Glode, J. E. and Wilson, C. B. (1974). Antitubular basement membrane antibodies in methicillin-associated interstitial nephritis. *N. Engl. J. Med.*, **291**, 381–384.

3. Kincaid-Smith, P. (1967). Pathogenesis of the renal lesions associated with the abuse of analgesics. *Lancet*, **1**, 859–862.

4. Abel, J. A. (1971). Analgesic nephropathy — review of the literature, 1967–70. *Clin. Pharmacol. Ther.*, **12**, 583–598.

5. Lagergren, C. and Ljungqvist, A. (1962). The international arterial pattern in renal papillary necrosis: A microangiographic and histological study. *Am. J. Pathol.*, **41**, 633–643.

6. Burry, A. F. (1968). The evolution of analgesic nephropathy. *Nephron*, **5**, 185–201.

7. Barnes, J. M., Austwick, P. K. C., Carter, R. L., Flynn, F. V., Peristianis, G. C. and Aldridge, W. N. (1977). Balkan (endemic) nephropathy and a toxin-producing strain of *Penicillium verrucosum* var. *cyclopium*: An experimental model in rats. *Lancet*, **1**, 671–675.

8. Spear, G. S. (1974). Pathology of the kidney in cystinosis. In Sommers, S. C. (ed.) *Pathology Annual*, Vol. 9, pp. 81–92. (New York: Appleton–Century–Croft).

Glomerulonephritis

8

The responses of the specialized capillaries of glomerular tufts to injury are in many ways analogous to those of capillaries elsewhere in the body. The range of resulting morphological changes, and the functional abnormalities produced, provide the structural and clinical expressions of what is collectively termed glomerulonephritis. Such changes may be primary or part of a systemic disease, but the initial damage to the kidney occurs in the glomeruli. Although tubular and interstitial lesions may also develop and are often extensive, these are regarded as secondary phenomena.

Whilst knowledge of the underlying aetiology and detailed pathogenesis of the various forms of glomerulonephritis is still far from complete, several advances during the last thirty years have improved our understanding. Many types of human glomerulonephritis appear to be immunologically mediated and our knowledge of these has been substantially facilitated by the development of appropriate animal models. The introduction of safe percutaneous renal biopsy techniques has permitted study of the evolution of human glomerulonephritis, and the correlation of the lesions found with the accompanying functional impairment and overall clinical course. Rapid fixation of biopsy specimens has provided improved morphological detail at the light microscopical level and the widespread use of ultrastructural analysis has greatly extended our knowledge of these structural changes. Plastic embedding of biopsy specimens from electron microscopy has provided a further advantage in that thin sections with a morphological clarity which is impossible to achieve by paraffin embedding techniques are available for light microscopy. With these plastic sections features hitherto only visible ultrastructurally can be distinguished with a conventional light microscope. The introduction of immunofluorescence microscopy has provided a further dimension to the study of renal biopsy specimens by permitting the localization of immunoglobulins and complement components within the glomeruli. This work is now being extended by immunoperoxidase techniques, which provide similar data in permanent preparations made from paraffin-embedded material which can be viewed by conventional light microscopes, or, with appropriate adaptation, at the ultrastructural level.

Two distinct immunological mechanisms have been identified in glomerulonephritis[1, 2].

(1) Fixation of anti-glomerular basement membrane antibodies to the glomerular basement membrane (anti-GBM disease), and

(2) Deposition of soluble immune (antibody–antigen) complexes from the circulation in the glomeruli (soluble complex disease).

In both forms, fixation and activation of the complement system is important in initiating glomerular damage and there is evidence that release of enzymes from neutrophil polymorphs and the activation of blood clotting mechanisms may also be involved.

Immunofluorescence or immunoperoxidase techniques are used to distinguish between the two mechanisms, anti-GBM disease being characterized by diffuse linear staining, outlining the glomerular basement membrane, whilst soluble complex disease causes a granular or 'lumpy-bumpy' staining either along the peripheral capillary loops, or within the mesangial regions, or both. Most human forms of glomerulonephritis appear on this basis to be soluble complex diseases, although Goodpasture's syndrome is well-documented as a form of anti-GBM disease[3].

One crucial factor determining whether or not glomerular trapping of circulating immune complexes occurs lies in their size. Dixon et al.[4] have shown that soluble complexes formed under conditions of moderate antigen excess are involved in initiating these forms of glomerulonephritis. Small complexes found in states of marked antigen excess remain in the circulation, and very large insoluble antigen–antibody aggregates formed in conditions of antibody excess are rapidly cleared from the circulation by the reticulo-endothelial system, so that glomerular trapping is normally a fleeting phenomenon. Soothill and Stewart[5] have suggested that complex size may be related to antibody affinity. Individuals who synthesize only low affinity antibodies, which bind antigen poorly, may produce circulating soluble complexes of relatively small size, capable of initiating soluble complex disease. If an impaired immune response of this nature is important in the genesis of immune complex disease, it may help to explain why glomerulonephritis is a relatively rare outcome in the presence of circulating complexes, and why immunosuppression is comparatively ineffective in the treatment of established disease. Variation of soluble complex size within the range capable of initiating glomerular injury may also help to explain some of the different morphological patterns of glomerulonephritis which occur. Germuth and Rodriguez[6] have provided experimental evidence that the smaller immune complexes are capable of penetrating the glomerular basement membrane, but become entrapped in the sub-epithelial space. This localization produces a different structural response from that elicited by larger complexes, which are held within the sub-endothelial space or the mesangium.

The different presenting clinical syndromes in patients suffering from glomerulonephritis give little indication of the nature of their disease or of its prognosis. For this reason, the classification of glomerulonephritis used is based on morphological considerations (see Table 8.1). The various types of glomerulonephritis are discussed in separate sections.

Table 8.1   Classification of glomerulonephritis

(1) Diffuse endocapillary proliferative glomerulonephritis
(2) Diffuse mesangial proliferative glomerulonephritis
(3) Diffuse mesangiocapillary glomerulonephritis
  (i) with sub-endothelial deposits
  (ii) with linear dense intra-membranous deposits
(4) Diffuse extracapillary glomerulonephritis
(5) Diffuse membranous glomerulonephritis
(6) 'Minimal change' disease
(7) Focal glomerulonephritis
  (i) Focal segmental proliferative glomerulonephritis
  (ii) Focal segmental/global glomerulosclerosis
(8) Diffuse global glomerulosclerosis

References

1. Unanue, E. R. and Dixon, F. J. (1967). Experimental glomerulonephritis: Immunological events and pathogenetic mechanisms. In Humphrey, J. and Dixon, F. J. (eds.), *Advances in Immunology*, Vol. 1, pp. 1–90. (New York: Academic Press).

2. Dixon, F. J. and Wilson, C. B. (1972). Immunological aspects of glomerulonephritis. In Black, D. (ed.) *Renal Disease*, 3rd Edn, pp. 275–294. (Oxford: Blackwell).

3. Wilson, C. B. and Dixon, F. J. (1973). Antiglomerular basement membrane antibody-induced glomerulonephritis. *Kidney Int.*, **3**, 74–89.

4. Dixon, F. J., Feldman, J. D. and Vazquez, J. J. (1961). Experimental glomerulonephritis. The pathogenesis of a laboratory model resembling the spectrum of human glomerulonephritis. *J. Exp. Med.*, **113**, 899–920.

5. Soothill, J. F. and Stewart M. V. (1971). The immunopathological significance of the heterogeneity of antibody affinity. *Clin. Exp. Immunol.*, **9**, 193–199.

6. Germuth, F. G. and Rodriguez, E. (1973). In *Immunopathology of the Renal Glomerulus*, pp. 81–91. (Boston: Little Brown and Co.).

9

Diffuse Endocapillary and Mesangial Proliferative Glomerulonephritis

Diffuse Endocapillary Proliferative Glomerulonephritis

Classically this form of glomerulonephritis follows infections with group A β-haemolytic streptococci (usually types 12, 4 or 1), and is regarded as a form of soluble complex disease developing during an immune reaction to the infecting organism. Clinical evidence of glomerulonephritis (haematuria, proteinuria, oliguria, hypocomplementaemia, facial oedema and often hypertension) presents acutely some 5–30 days after the streptococcal infection. The patients are often children or young adults. Cases are usually sporadic but may occasionally occur in epidemics as, for example, the Red Lake incident in North America, which followed an outbreak of streptococcal skin infection[1].

On light microscopy during the acute phase the most conspicuous feature is a marked hypercellularity affecting all the glomerular tufts (Figure 9.1). The glomerular tufts are swollen, filling the urinary spaces, and show accentuated lobulation. The hypercellularity is due largely to a proliferation of endocapillary (mesangial and endothelial) cells and is usually sufficient to occlude many of the capillary loops. Recent studies[2] suggest that the majority of the proliferating cells are modified mesangial cells which extend into the capillary loops beneath the endothelium. Frequently, the tufts are infiltrated by varying numbers of neutrophil polymorphs (Figure 9.2). Immunochemical techniques reveal coarse granular deposits of immunoglobulins (principally IgG) and C3 in a mainly peripheral distribution in the glomerular tufts (Figure 9.3). Ultrastructurally, dense deposits (regarded as aggregates of immune complexes) are seen mainly in the sub-epithelial space, but also occasionally beneath the endothelium and in the mesangium. Very large sub-epithelial deposits ('humps') are characteristic and can often be seen by light microscopy in 1μm sections of plastic-embedded tissue (Figures 9.4, 9.5 and 9.6). Identification of streptococcal antigens in the deposits has proved difficult, but Treser et al.[3] have shown by immunofluorescence microscopy that convalescent serum from patients recovering from post-streptococcal glomerulonephritis binds to the glomeruli in biopsies taken from the same patients during the acute phase. This activity could be abolished by absorption of the sera with plasma membrane preparations from certain types of group A streptococci.

In the majority of patients, particularly children, the disease is short-lived and complete clinical recovery is the rule, although a small proportion may progress to chronic renal failure after a number of years[4, 5]. Sub-epithelial 'humps' are not usually seen by electron microscopy in biopsies taken more than six weeks after onset in patients who subsequently recover. Deposits of C3 sometimes persist in the mesangial regions for many months and this is associated with some residual mesangial hypercellularity, although the peripheral capillary loops return to normal.

The severity of the glomerular changes varies from case to case. Epithelial cell proliferation with capsular crescent formation (see diffuse extracapillary GN) may occur in some glomeruli and if extensive may be associated with acute renal failure, requiring dialysis (Figures 9.7 and 9.8). However, even in these cases appropriate treatment is usually followed by clinical recovery although some degree of residual glomerular and interstitial scarring is generally apparent on subsequent biopsies (Figure 9.9).

Diffuse endocapillary proliferative glomerulonephritis is often regarded as synonymous with acute post-streptococcal glomerulonephritis, but this is not entirely accurate. Increasingly in recent years evidence of a preceding streptococcal infection has become uncommon in patients with this type of glomerulonephritis[6], and, furthermore, streptococcal infections may occasionally be followed by other types of glomerulonephritis, notably the mesangiocapillary form. Patients with infected ventriculo-atrial shunts inserted for the relief of hydrocephalus may develop diffuse glomerulonephritis of either endocapillary proliferative or mesangiocapillary patterns. These cases provide concrete examples of non-streptococcal antigens which may be associated with these forms of glomerulonephritis.

Diffuse Mesangial Proliferative Glomerulonephritis

This is a non-specific pattern of glomerulonephritis characterized on light microscopy by a diffuse expansion of the mesangial regions of the glomerular tufts by a combination of mesangial cell proliferation and an increase in mesangial matrix seen particularly well in sections stained by the PAS method. An important feature is that the cellular proliferation is insufficiently marked to cause significant occlusion of the capillary loops, the walls of which appear normal (Figures 9.10 and 9.11).

Mesangial proliferative glomerulonephritis is a fairly common glomerular reaction seen both as an isolated renal lesion and as part of several systemic diseases. Its evaluation depends on the associated clinical features and information gained by immunochemical techniques and electron microscopy.

In the absence of systemic disease mesangial proliferative glomerulonephritis may be associated clinically with the nephrotic syndrome or the recurrent haematuria syndrome. Affected patients are usually children or young adults. An indistinguishable histological pattern is also seen in some patients

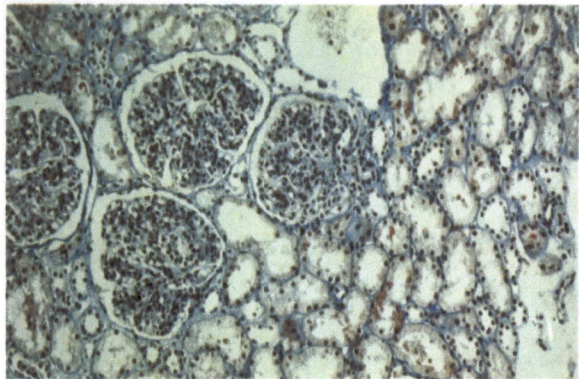

Figure 9.1 Diffuse endocapillary proliferative glomerulonephritis (DEPG). All the glomerular tufts are hypercellular and the glomerular capillary lumina inconspicuous. MSB   ×240.

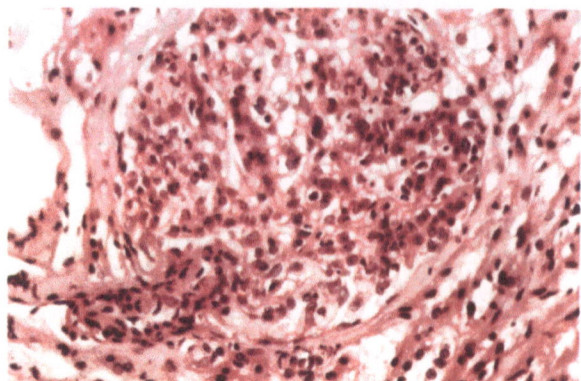

Figure 9.2 DEPG. The glomerular tuft is enlarged and fills the urinary space. The endocapillary cell proliferation obliterates many capillary lumina and in places neutrophil polymorphs can be seen infiltrating the tuft. H & E   ×720.

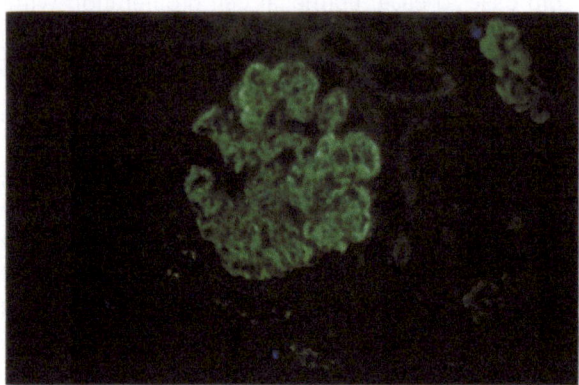

Figure 9.3 DEPG. Immunofluorescence microscopy showing coarse deposits of C3 predominantly on the capillary wall at the periphery of the tuft.   ×240.

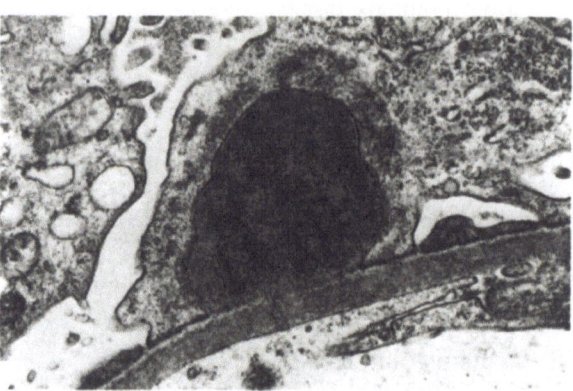

Figure 9.4 DEPG. An electron micrograph of a large electron-dense deposit ('hump') situated on the external aspect of the glomerular basement membrane (sub-epithelial deposit). There is 'fusion' of the foot processes of the overlying epithelial-cell.   ×15 000.

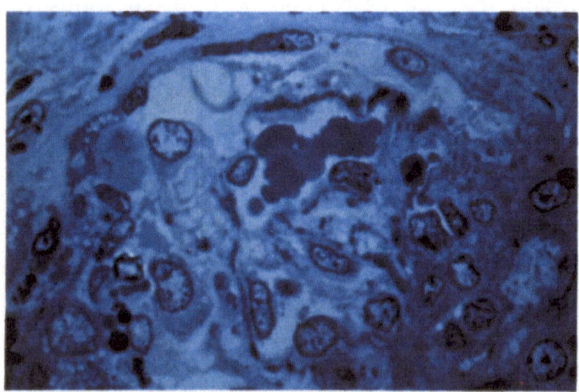

Figure 9.5 DEPG. Thin (1 μm) plastic-embedded section of part of a glomerular tuft showing conspicuous sub-epithelial deposits corresponding with those seen ultrastructurally (see Figure 9.4). Toluidine blue ×1440.

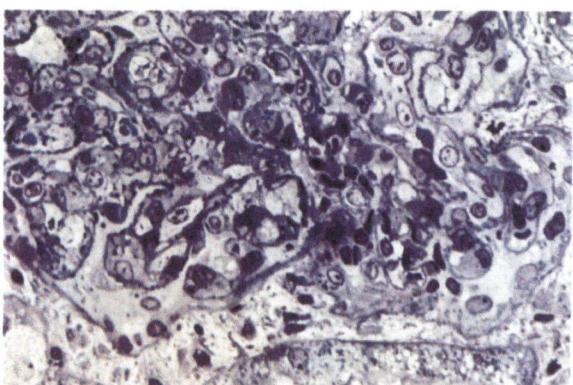

Figure 9.6 DEPG. Thin (1 μm) plastic-embedded section of part of a glomerular tuft with not only sub-epithelial but also sub-endothelial and occasional mesangial deposits. Toluidine blue   ×960.

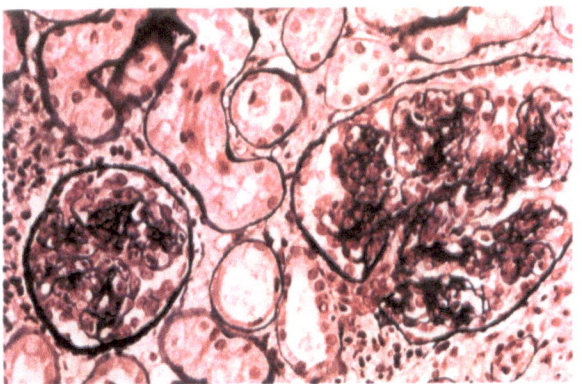

Figure 9.7   First biopsy from a case of acute post-streptococcal glomerulonephritis in a female child, aged nine years. This shows classical diffuse endocapillary proliferative glomerulonephritis. Methenamine silver/ H & E   × 480.

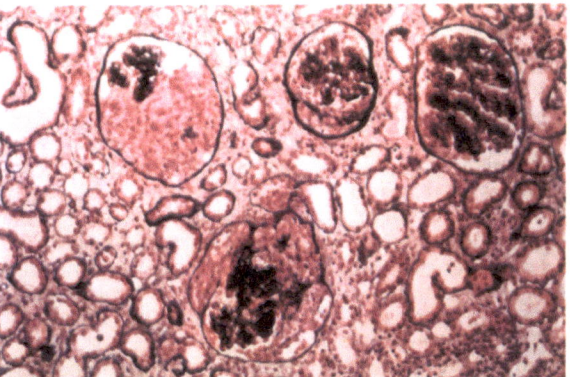

Figure 9.8   Second biopsy from the same case (Figure 9.7) taken 7 days later when the child had developed acute renal failure. This shows large epithelial crescents in 75% of glomeruli. Methenamine silver/H & E × 240.

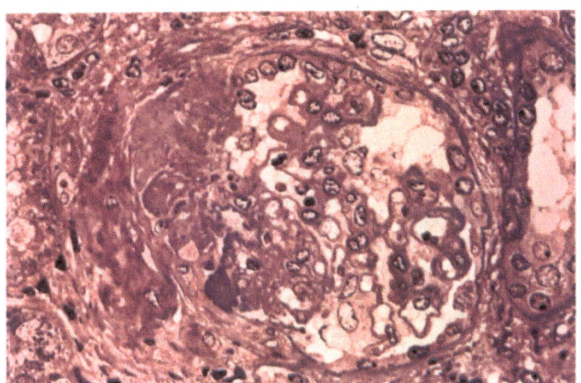

Figure 9.9   Third biopsy from the same case (Figures 9.7 and 9.8) taken 12 months later when the child was clinically well. Some glomeruli show segmental sclerosis. Toluidine blue plastic-embedded section   × 720.

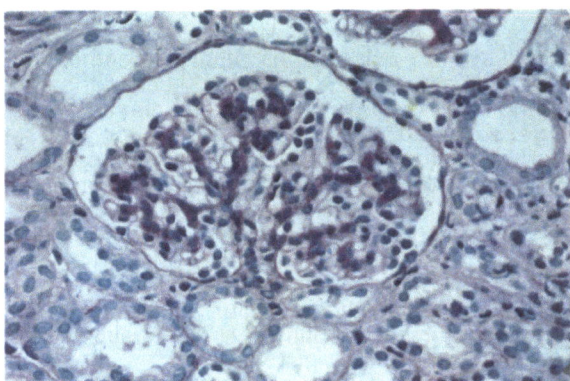

Figure 9.10   Diffuse mesangial proliferative glomerulonephritis. A glomerular tuft showing an increase in mesangial matrix and hypercellularity confined to mesangial regions. There is no capillary wall thickening and the peripheral capillary lumina are widely patent. PAS   × 480.

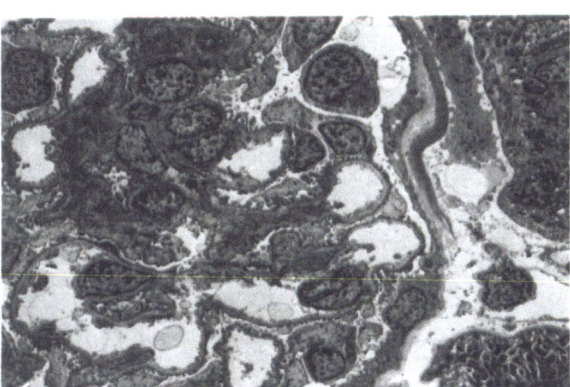

Figure 9.11   An electron micrograph showing mild residual mesangial hypercellularity in a case of resolving post-streptococcal glomerulonephritis; deposits are absent at this stage.   × 2400.

during the resolving phase following diffuse endo-capillary proliferative glomerulonephritis[7].

Patients with the nephrotic syndrome associated with mesangial proliferative glomerulonephritis do not usually respond to steroid therapy, and such treatment is generally contra-indicated since spontaneous clinical and histological resolution occur in the majority of cases. Immunochemical techniques are often entirely negative although occasionally mesangial deposits of immunoglobulins (usually IgA) and C3 are found.

Patients with recurrent haematuria and mesangial proliferative glomerulonephritis often have mesangial deposits of IgA, sometimes with IgG, and C3. Ultrastructurally, dense deposits are visible in the mesangium and often particularly large deposits occur at the edges of the mesangium against the adjacent capillary basement membrane. These deposits occasionally encroach upon the sub-endothelial space and elicit a segmental proliferation of mesangial cells which partially occlude the capillary lumens. When sufficiently large, these 'paramesangial' deposits may be visible by light microscopy, particularly in $1\mu m$ sections of plastic-embedded tissue. The association of recurrent haematuria and mesangial IgA deposition is often referred to as Berger's disease[8]. The original description is of a focal segmental proliferative glomerulonephritis, but further experience suggests that the segmental pattern is superimposed on a diffuse mesangial proliferative response as described above. Berger's disease cannot be used as a synonym for IgA nephropathy since not all patients with the recurrent haematuria syndrome exhibit a mesangial proliferative glomerulonephritis and equally some patients with IgA nephropathy present other than with recurrent haematuria.

Systemic diseases which may be associated with mesangial proliferative glomerulonephritis include Henoch–Schönlein disease (anaphylactoid purpura), systemic lupus erythematosus, Alport's syndrome and cirrhosis of the liver.

References

1. Kleinman, H. (1954). Epidemic acute glomerulonephritis at Red Lake. *Minn. Med. J.*, **37**, 479–483.

2. Thomson, K. and Turner, D. R. (1976). Mesangial cell cytoplasm and glomerular disease. *J. Pathol.*, **120**, 229–234.

3. Treser, G., Semar, M., Ty, A., Sagel, I., Franklin, M. A. and Lange, K. (1970). Partial characterization of antigenic streptococcal plasma membrane components in acute glomerulonephritis. *J. Clin. Invest.*, **49**, 762–768.

4. Baldwin, D. S., Gluck, M. C., Schacht, R. G. and Gallo, G. R. (1974). The long-term course of poststreptococcal glomerulonephritis. *Ann. Int. Med.*, **80**, 342–358.

5. Schacht, R. G., Gluck, M. C., Gallo, G. R. and Baldwin, D. S. (1976). Progression to uremia after remission of acute poststreptococcal glomerulonephritis. *N. Engl. J. Med.*, **295**, 977–981.

6. Meadow, S. R. (1975). Poststreptococcal nephritis — a rare disease. *Arch. Dis. Child.*, **50**, 379–382.

7. Jennings, R. B. and Earle, D. P. (1961). Poststreptococcal glomerulonephritis: Histopathologic and clinical studies of acute, subsiding acute and early chronic latent phases. *J. Clin. Invest.*, **40**, 1525–1595.

8. Berger, J., Yaneva, H. and Hinglais, N. (1971). Immunochemistry of glomerulonephritis. In Hamberger, J., Crosnier, J. and Maxwell, M. H. (eds.), *Advances in Nephrology*, Vol. 1, pp. 11–30. (Chicago: Yearbook Medical Publishers).

Diffuse Mesangiocapillary and Extracapillary Proliferative Glomerulonephritis

Diffuse Mesangiocapillary Glomerulonephritis

In this variety of glomerulonephritis (also termed membrano-proliferative glomerulonephritis), the glomeruli are uniformly involved, the tufts are enlarged and show prominent. lobulation. A variable proliferation of mesangial cells and increase in the amount of mesangial matrix is associated with diffuse thickening of glomerular capillary walls. This form of glomerulonephritis usually presents with an acute nephritic syndrome followed by a nephrotic syndrome which progresses over a number of years to chronic renal failure (Figure 10.1).

Although uncommon, mesangiocapillary glomerulonephritis is an important cause of renal failure in older children and young adults[1]. More than half the patients have persistently low serum C3 levels, and in these a C3 nephritic factor can generally be demonstrated (see below). As the disease progresses, hyalinization of the mesangial regions of glomerular tufts associated with diminished hypercellularity may occur giving an appearance which may be confused with diabetic nephropathy (see Chapter 15), and accounting for its older description as 'chronic lobular glomerulonephritis'[2]. Ultrastructurally, the capillary wall thickening may be of two main types and cases are classified on this basis[3, 4].

'Double Contour' or 'Sub-endothelial Deposit' Variety

Capillary wall thickening is due to the extension of mesangial cells around the circumference of the capillary loop, interposed between the basement membrane and the lining endothelium. A second layer of basement membrane-like material is formed between the mesangial layer and the endothelium, which can be demonstrated on light microscopy by silver methenamine impregnation giving a 'double contour' or 'tram-line' appearance (Figure 10.2). Electron, and sometimes light, microscopy can be used to identify deposited material along the endothelial aspect of the glomerular basement membrane, and often in the mesangium (Figures 10.3 and 10.4). Immunochemical techniques identify C3 and often immunoglobulins along the capillary loops and usually in the mesangium (Figure 10.5).

The 'sub-endothelial deposit' variety of mesangiocapillary glomerulonephritis may exceptionally follow streptococcal infections although usually no predisposing cause can be demonstrated. However, an identical morphology may be seen in nephritis associated with infected ventriculo-atrial shunts, infective endocarditis and plasmodium malarial infections[5]; rarely glomerulonephritis complicating systemic lupus erythematosus or Henoch–Schönlein disease is of this type.

'Linear Dense Deposit' Variety

In this rarer form of mesangiocapillary glomerulonephritis, capillary wall thickening is due to a ribbon-like deposit within the basement membrane itself. Similar deposits frequently occur in the basement membranes of Bowman's capsule and the renal tubules. Ultrastructurally, the deposit is intensely electron-dense and replaces the lamina densa (Figure 10.6). It is seen well in thin sections of plastic-embedded material, stained with toluidine blue for which it has a high affinity (Figure 10.7). By light microscopy it stains intensely with PAS but is not argyrophilic (Figure 10.8). This is a useful point, since mesangial cell proliferation is often not conspicuous and may lead to a mistaken diagnosis of membranous glomerulonephritis. Not uncommonly in this variety of glomerular disease, a proportion of glomeruli contain epithelial crescents. Immunochemical techniques reveal deposits of C3 only (Figure 10.9). These are mainly in the mesangium with weak or negative staining of the capillary loops.

Low serum complement levels in mesangiocapillary glomerulonephritis are due partly to diminished synthesis and partly to the presence of a serum factor (C3 nephritic factor) which causes consumption of complement via the alternative pathway[6]. Mesangiocapillary glomerulonephritis of the 'linear dense' variety may also be associated with partial lipodystrophy[7]. Patients with partial lipodystrophy and mesangiocapillary glomerulonephritis almost invariably exhibit hypocomplementaemia and occasionally the hypocomplementaemia may precede evidence of glomerulonephritis by some years. Transplantation in patients with the linear dense deposit variety is associated with a high recurrence rate in the graft[8].

Diffuse Extracapillary Proliferative Glomerulonephritis

This term encompasses any glomerulonephritis in which there is marked proliferation of extracapillary cells (i.e. cells outside the glomerular capillary basement membrane) causing obliteration of the urinary space (so-called 'capsular crescent' formation) and affecting at least 80% of unsclerosed glomeruli. This extracapillary cell proliferation is often so marked that the associated glomerular tuft is compressed and obscured. The glomerular tuft may show no significant changes beyond compression,

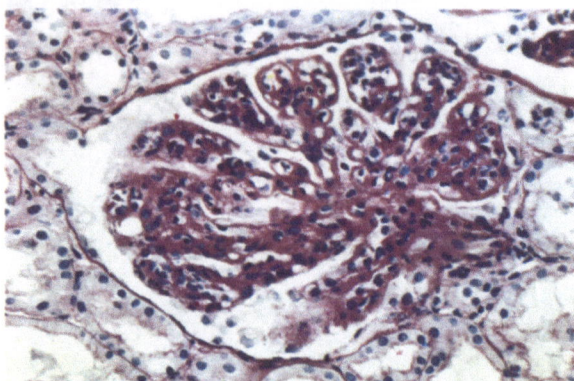

Figure 10.1 Mesangiocapillary glomerulonephritis. The glomerulus is enlarged and shows accentuated lobulation of the tuft. There is both diffuse thickening of the walls of tuft capillary loops and mesangial cell proliferation. PAS × 480.

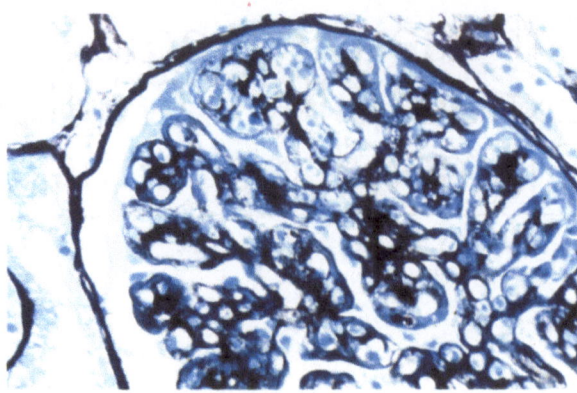

Figure 10.2 Mesangiocapillary glomerulonephritis ('double contour' variety). A silver methenamine preparation showing widespread 'tramlining' of the capillary loops. This change is not always as extensive as illustrated here and may require a careful search of a well stained section with an oil-immersion objective for its demonstration. × 960.

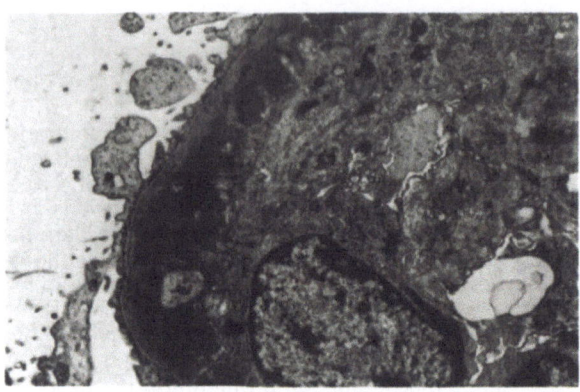

Figure 10.3 Mesangiocapillary glomerulonephritis ('double contour' variety). An electron micrograph showing large sub-endothelial deposits and interposition of mesangial cell cytoplasm beneath the endothelium. This virtually obliterates the capillary lumen. × 8200.

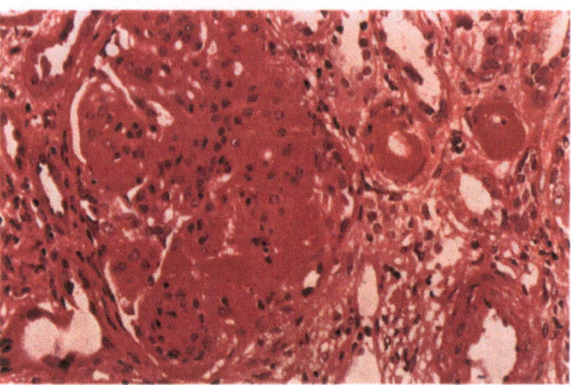

Figure 10.4 Mesangiocapillary glomerulonephritis ('double contour' variety). A paraffin section stained by PAS showing magenta-staining sub-endothelial deposits both in the lower part of the glomerular tuft and in the adjacent afferent arteriole. × 480.

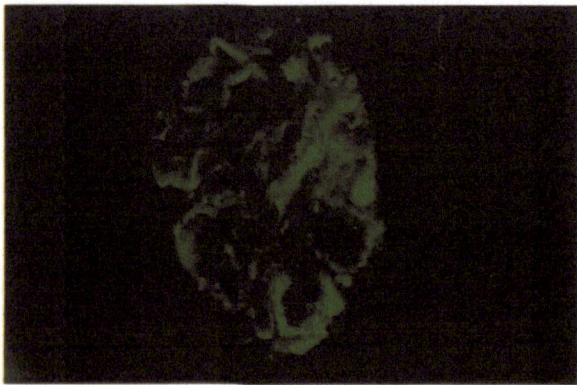

Figure 10.5 Mesangiocapillary glomerulonephritis. Immunofluorescence microscopy showing immunoglobulin deposition mainly along the capillary loops. × 360.

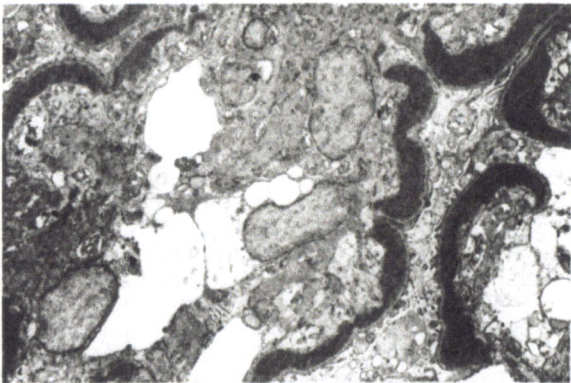

Figure 10.6 Mesangiocapillary glomerulonephritis (dense deposit variety). An electron micrograph showing a ribbon-like dense deposit within the basement membrane. Mesangial cell proliferation is mild. × 4880.

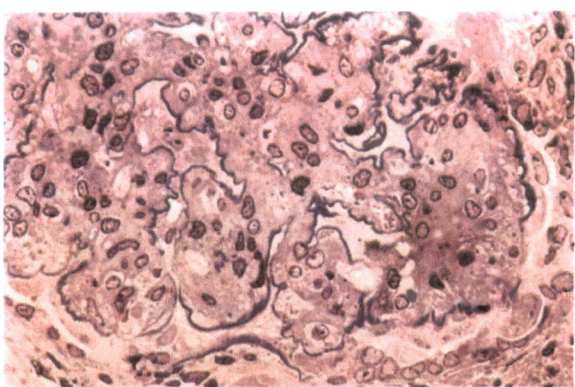

Figure 10.7   Mesangiocapillary glomerulonephritis (dense deposit variety). The linear dense deposits are stained intensely with toluidine blue in this plastic-embedded section.   × 960.

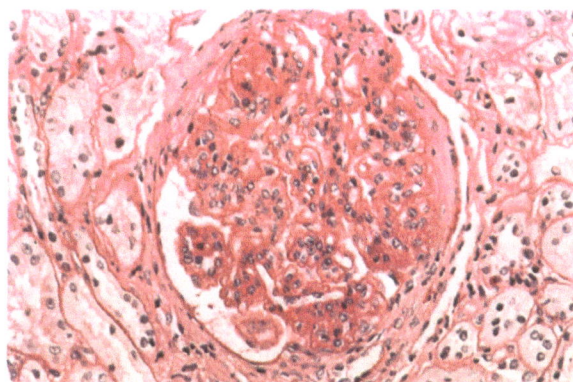

Figure 10.8   Mesangiocapillary glomerulonephritis (dense deposit variety). A paraffin-embedded section showing intense staining of the linear deposits with PAS. These deposits are non-argyrophilic with methenamine silver which is a useful point of differentiation. PAS   × 480.

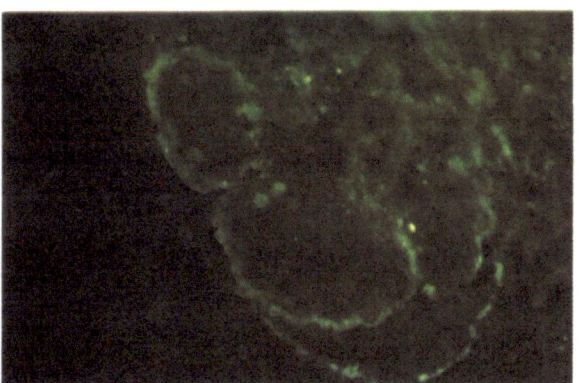

Figure 10.9   Mesangiocapillary glomerulonephritis (linear dense deposit variety). Immunofluorescence microscopy showing deposition of C3 along the glomerular capillary loops. Immunoglobulin deposition is not a feature of this condition.   × 960.

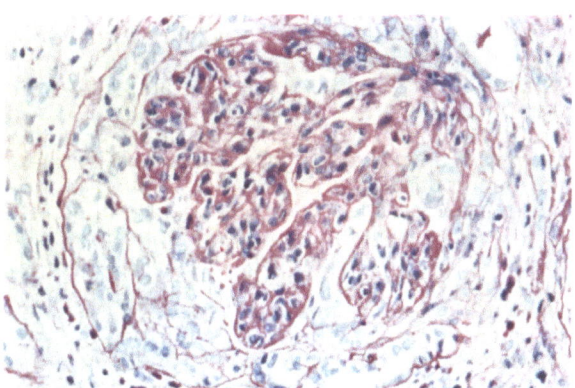

Figure 10.10   Extracapillary proliferative glomerulonephritis. The glomerular tuft showing accentuated lobulation and hypercellularity. There is conspicuous proliferation of extracapillary cells which fill the urinary space to form a 'capsular crescent'. PAS   × 600.

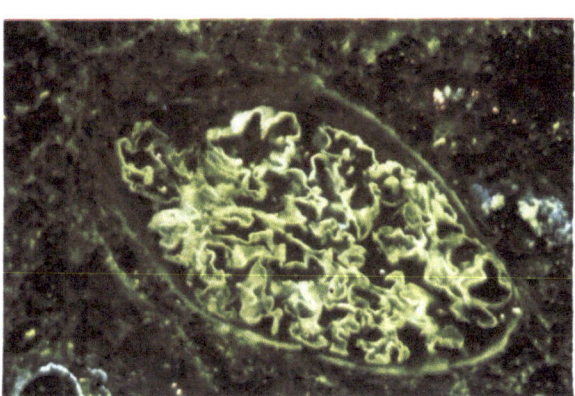

Figure 10.11   Goodpasture's syndrome. Immunofluorescence microscopy showing linear staining of the glomerular capillary basement membrane for IgG, indicating anti-GBM disease.   × 480.

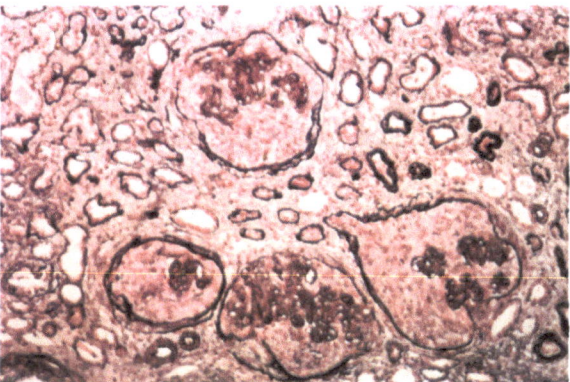

Figure 10.12   Diffuse extracapillary proliferative glomerulonephritis. Four glomeruli showing conspicuous capsular crescents. This biopsy is from a patient with mesangiocapillary glomerulonephritis and illustrates the essentially non-specific character of capsular crescent formation. Methenamine silver/H & E   × 240.

or there may be evidence of other patterns of glomerulonephritis such as endocapillary or mesangiocapillary proliferative glomerulonephritis (Figures 10.10 and 10.12). A variable pattern of glomerular tuft proliferation may suggest a pre-existing focal segmental proliferative glomerulonephritis, associated with systemic disease such as Henoch–Schönlein disease or systemic lupus erythematosus.

Goodpasture's syndrome, the only well-documented form of human anti-GBM disease, may also be associated with diffuse extracapillary proliferative glomerulonephritis (Figure 10.11).

Thus this glomerular lesion is quite non-specific both in terms of underlying pathogenic mechanisms and associated disease. The justification for its separate classification lies in its generally grave prognostic significance reflected in the older term 'rapidly progressive glomerulonephritis' used to describe it. The widespread obliteration of glomerular urinary spaces by capsular crescents severely compromises urine production and often results in acute renal failure.

The marked extracapillary cellular proliferation is believed to represent a reaction to leakage of fibrin into the urinary space. The proliferating cells are traditionally regarded as epithelial cells derived from those covering the glomerular tuft and lining Bowman's capsule, although recent studies[9] suggest that macrophages derived from circulating monocytes may be an important component of the crescents. Because fibrin deposition appears to be important in precipitating capsular crescent formation and because the outlook for affected patients is so poor, intensive treatment has been instituted in some centres which includes the use of anticoagulant and fibrinolytic agents. Such therapies occasionally result in dramatic improvements[10, 11]

References

1. West, C. D., McAdams, A. J., McConville, J. M., Davis, N. C. and Holland, N. H. (1965). Hypocomplementemic and normocomplementemic persistent (chronic) glomerulonephritis; clinical and pathologic characteristics. *J. Paediatr.*, **67**, 1089–1112.

2. Heptinstall, R. H. (1974). Lobular glomerulonephritis. In *Pathology of the Kidney*, 2nd Edn, pp. 425–432. (Boston: Little, Brown and Co.).

3. Berger, J. and Galle, P. (1963). Dépôts denses au sein des membranes basales du rein. Étude en microscopie optique et électronique. *Presse Med.*, **71**, 2351–2354.

4. Levy, M., Loirat, C. and Habib, R. (1973). Idiopathic membrano-proliferative glomerulonephritis in children (correlations between light, electron, immunofluorescent microscopic appearances and serum C3 and C4 levels). *Biomed. Express*, **19**, 447–454.

5. Tighe, J. R. (1975). Nephrotic syndrome and quartan malaria. In Harrison, C. V. and Weinbren, K. (ed.) *Recent Advances in Pathology*, Vol. 9, pp. 147–155. (Edinburgh: Churchill Livingstone).

6. Spitzer, R. E., Vallota, E. H., Forristal, J., Sudora, E., Stitzel, A., Davïs, N. C. and West, C. D. (1969). Serum C3 lytic system in patients with glomerulonephritis. *Science*, **164**, 436–437.

7. Peters, D. K., Williams, D. C., Charlesworth, J. A., Boulton-Jones, J. M., Sissons, J. G. P., Evans, D. J., Kourilsky, O. and Moret-Maroger, L. (1973). Mesangiocapillary nephritis, partial lipodystrophy and hypocomplementaemia. *Lancet*, **2**, 535–538.

8. Turner, D. R., Cameron, J. S., Bewick, M., Sharpstone, P., Melcher, D., Ogg, C. S., Evans, D. J., Trafford, A. J. P. and Leibowitz, S. (1976). Transplantation in mesangiocapillary glomerulonephritis with intramembranous dense deposits: recurrence of disease. *Kidney Int.*, **9**, 439–448.

9. Atkins, R. C., Holdsworth, S. R., Glasgow, E. F. and Mathews, E. F. (1976). The macrophage in human rapidly progressive glomerulonephritis. *Lancet*, **1**, 830–832.

10. Brown, C. B., Wilson, D., Turner, D. R., Cameron, J. S., Ogg, C. S., Chantler, C. and Gill, D. (1974). Combined immunosuppresion and anti-coagulation in rapidly progressive glomerulonephritis. *Lancet*, **2**, 1166–1172.

11. Lockwood, C. M., Pinching, A. J., Sweny, P., Rees, A. J., Pussell, B., Uff, J. and Peters, D. K. (1977). Plasma-exchange and immunosuppression in the treatment of fulminating immune complex crescentic nephritis. *Lancet*, **1**, 63–67.

Diffuse Membranous Glomerulonephritis and 'Minimal Change' Disease

Diffuse Membranous Glomerulonephritis

This type of glomerulonephritis is characterized histologically by diffuse thickening of the walls of all glomerular capillaries without significant cellular proliferation (Figure 11.1). Some mesangial prominence is occasionally present[1] and in such cases the possibility of lupus nephritis should be excluded (see page 58). Electron microscopy, or the use of special techniques such as silver methenamine impregnation (Figure 11.2) or trichrome stains, or thin sections of plastic-embedded tissue examined by light microscopy, show that the glomerular capillary wall thickening is due primarily to discrete deposits closely applied to the epithelial aspect of the glomerular basement membrane (Figure 11.3). Ehrenreich and Churg[2] have traced the evolution of the glomerular lesion and have shown that, as the lesion progresses, spike-like extensions of the glomerular basement membrane protrude between the deposits like the teeth of a comb (Figure 11.4). The formation of more basement membrane material continues until eventually the deposits are surrounded. The deposits ultimately become less distinct as they are incorporated into the now greatly thickened basement membrane (Figure 11.5). Collapse and obliteration of affected capillary loops result in the gradual hyalinization of whole glomeruli. Immunochemical techniques reveal a characteristic beaded pattern along the glomerular capillary loops of deposits containing C3 and IgG, and sometimes IgM and IgA (Figures 11.6, 11.7 and 11.8). In very early membranous nephropathy, capillary wall thickening may be only focal or inapparent. At this stage the change is easily missed by light microscopy and an erroneous diagnosis of 'minimal change' disease can result. Immunochemical techniques will nevertheless show a typical beaded pattern and deposits can usually be identified by electron microscopy.

Patients with this type of glomerulonephritis usually present clinically with proteinuria which is generally heavy and associated with the nephrotic syndrome. Response to steroid therapy is unusual. All ages may be affected, although the lesion is commoner in adults. A gradual progression to chronic renal failure over a period of years is usual, although temporary remissions and even spontaneous clinical and histological resolution may occur (Figure 11.9), and this appears to be commoner in children[3]. This form of glomerulonephropathy may be produced in animal models and is usually regarded as a form of chronic immune complex disease. Evans[4] has suggested that the epithelial deposits might result from precipitation of soluble precursors (antigen and antibody), which have diffused through the basement membrane and become concentrated in the sub-endothelial space.

Assuming an equilibrium between these precipitates and their soluble precursors, resorption of the deposits might occur following dissociation due to changing antigen—antibody balance, and so explain the occasional resolution of the lesion. The lack of mesangial cell proliferation is usually explained by the position of the deposits outside the basement membrane and the lack of immune complexes within the mesangium.

In most human cases of membranous nephritis, the underlying cause is unknown although occasionally the responsible antigenic stimulus can be identified. This pattern of glomerular disease may follow treatment with some drugs (gold and penicillamine), chronic hepatitis-associated antigenaemia and the presence of some malignant tumours (particularly carcinoma of the bronchus). In some cases of lupus nephritis, membranous transformation may occur, and although this appearance is usually part of a 'mixed' glomerulonephritis with accompanying deposits and cellular proliferation in the mesangium, occasionally a 'pure' membranous glomerulonephritis may be seen.

'Minimal Change' Disease

It has been recognized for many years that the majority of children (more than 80%), and a minority of adults (about 10%), who present with the nephrotic syndrome show an absence of, or only trivial, glomerular changes by light microscopy (Figures 11.10 and 11.11). Glomerular deposition of immunoglobulins, complement or fibrin is nearly always absent by immunochemical techniques, although a small minority of cases has been reported in which some mainly mesangial IgA, IgG and IgM deposition has been noted. In untreated cases, diffuse fusion and coalescence of epithelial foot processes is seen by electron microscopy (Figure 11.12), but this is usually regarded as a consequence rather than a cause of the heavy proteinuria[5]. Other secondary changes are usually seen in the renal tubular cells, such as hyaline droplet change which also reflects massive proteinuria, and prominent lipid deposition, a consequence of deranged lipid metabolism seen in the nephrotic syndrome, and responsible for the older term of 'lipoid nephrosis' used to describe this condition[6,7].

The pathogenesis of 'minimal change' disease has yet to be established. Evidence for underlying immunological mechanisms such as changes in the levels of serum immunoconglutinin and complement is indirect evidence of the involvement of immunological mechanisms[8] but the generally negative immunochemical findings are against the concept that glomerular immune complex deposition is

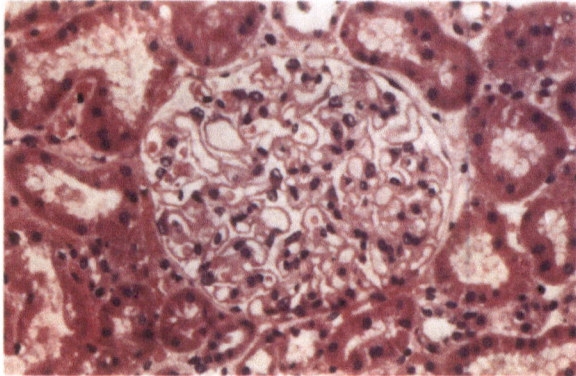

Figure 11.1 Membranous glomerulonephritis. The glomerular capillary walls are diffusely and uniformly thickened. There is no significant cellular proliferation. H & E × 600.

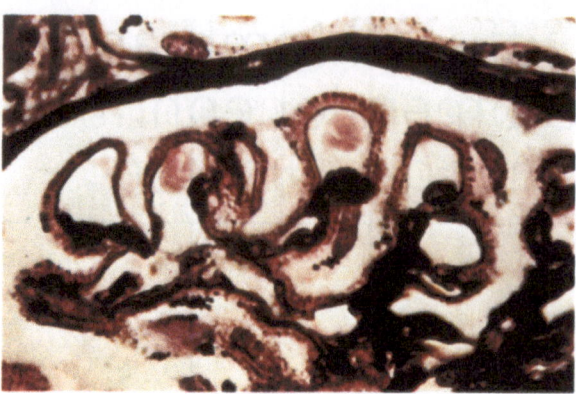

Figure 11.2 Membranous glomerulonephritis. Part of a glomerular tuft impregnated with methenamine silver to illustrate the 'spikes' of argyrophilic material extending outwards from the external aspect of the glomerular capillary basement membranes. As here, these 'spikes' often have expanded, 'knob-like' ends.   × 1400.

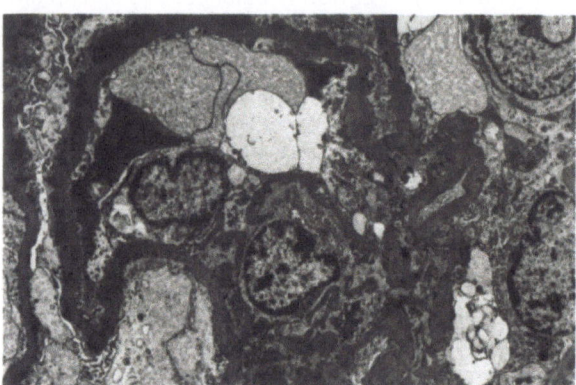

Figure 11.3 Membranous glomerulonephritis (early stage). An electron micrograph illustrating electron-dense, sub-epithelial deposits with associated focal 'fusion' of foot-processes but little change in the basement membrane.   × 3640.

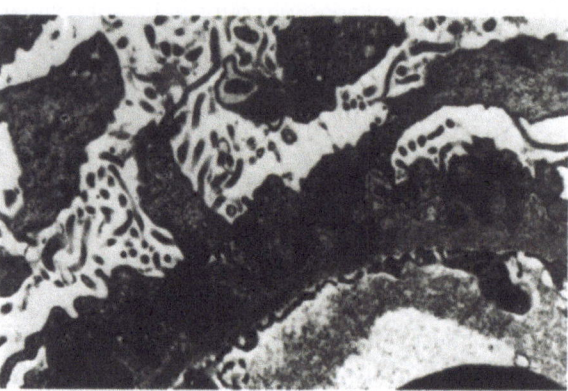

Figure 11.4 Membranous glomerulonephritis (established). An electron micrograph showing more numerous sub-epithelial deposits (cf. Figure 11.3) and extensions of basement membrane material between them. Foot-process 'fusion' is more generalized.   × 6600.

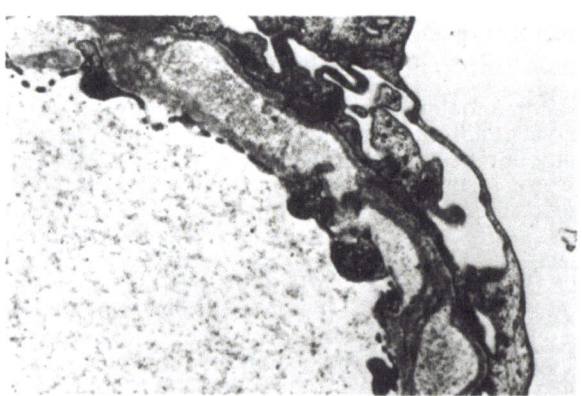

Figure 11.5 Membranous glomerulonephritis in late stage. Lucent areas are present within the greatly thickened basement membrane and are thought to represent sites previously occupied by deposits.   × 9600.

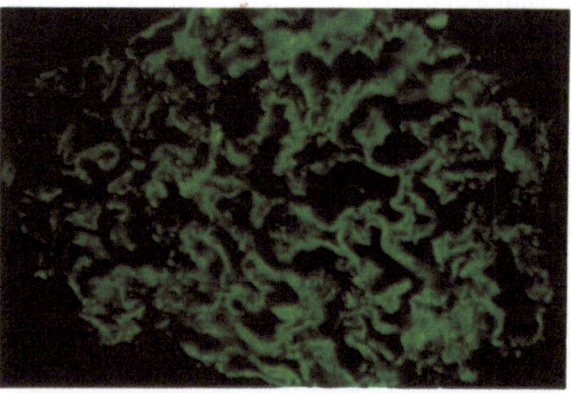

Figure 11.6 Membranous glomerulonephritis. Immunofluorescence microscopy showing diffuse deposition of immunoglobulin (IgG along the capillary loops but sparing the mesangium).   × 960.

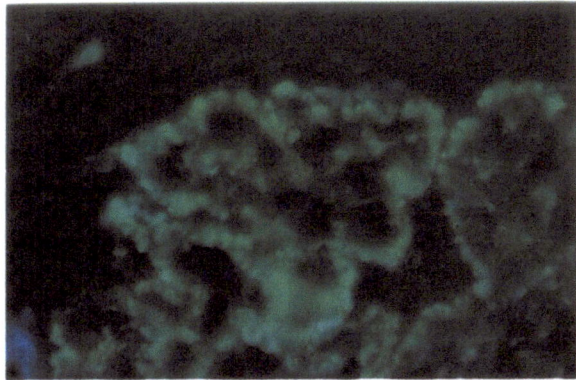

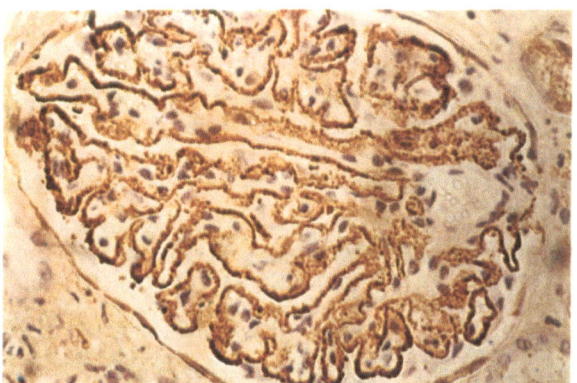

Figure 11.7 Membranous glomerulonephritis. High power of the same glomerulus illustrated in Figure 11.6, showing the granular, 'beaded' character of the deposits of IgG. ×1400.

Figure 11.8 Membranous glomerulonephritis. Immunoperoxidase staining of a paraffin section for IgG. ×960.

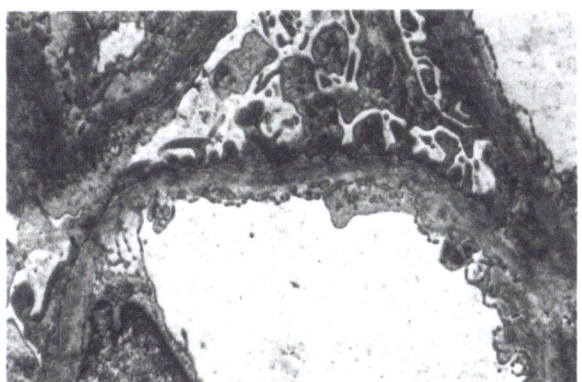

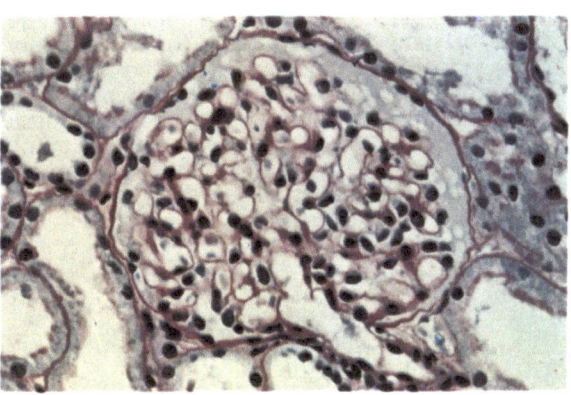

Figure 11.9 Membranous glomerulonephritis with resolution. A 40-year-old woman developed membranous glomerulonephritis following penicillamine treatment for rheumatoid arthritis. Therapy was stopped when proteinuria was noted. The amount of protein in her urine gradually diminished over the next 10 months. When the biopsy illustrated here was taken at the end of this period, the glomerular basement membrane showed only minor irregularities of its sub-epithelial aspect without electron dense deposits. ×4800.

Figure 11.10 'Minimal change' disease. A glomerulus showing no obvious abnormality to light microscopy, from a biopsy taken from a 4-year-old boy with steroid-sensitive nephrotic syndrome. PAS ×600.

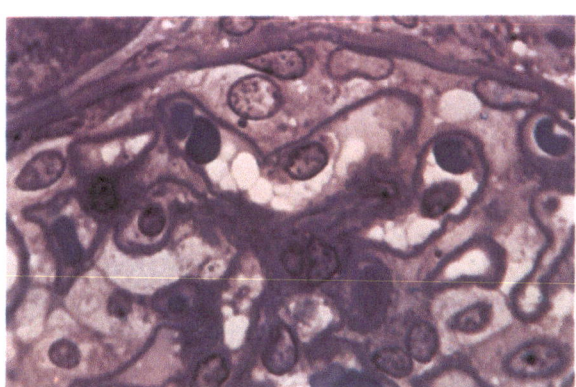

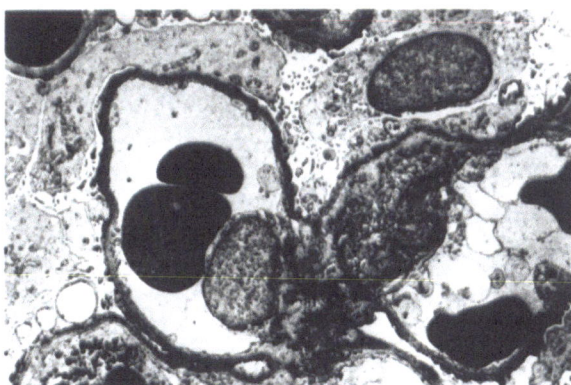

Figure 11.11 'Minimal change' disease. A plastic-embedded section of part of a glomerulus showing the absence of significant morphological abnormality. Toluidine blue ×1400:

Figure 11.12 'Minimal change' disease. An electron micrograph of part of the glomerulus in an untreated case, showing widespread 'fusion' of foot-processes. The cytoplasm of epithelial podocytes in many areas is in direct continuity with basement membrane. ×3600.

involved. The possibility that lymphokines secreted by lymphocytes in a cell-mediated hypersensitivity reaction might be involved in production of proteinuria in minimal change disease has been suggested by Lagrue *et al*[9].

The peak incidence of minimal change disease with the nephrotic syndrome is in children between 2 and 4 years of age and boys are affected three times as often as girls. The proteinuria is usually highly selective (i.e. the urinary protein is predominantly albumen), and is not accompanied by haematuria. Characteristically, treatment with high dose of steroids results in complete loss of proteinuria and reversion of the epithelial foot process fusion. About 20% of children have only one or two nephrotic episodes before going into permanent remission. The remainder relapse after a shorter or longer period when steroid therapy is withdrawn. In about half of these patients relapse occurs almost immediately when steroids are stopped and this 'frequently relapsing steroid-sensitive' group poses a difficult clinical problem, particularly as large dosages of steroid are required. More satisfactory remissions can sometimes be achieved with immunosuppressive drugs, such as cyclophosphamide.[10] However, the longterm effects of these drugs, particularly on the gonads, has yet to be established. Despite the marked tendency for patients with minimal change disease to relapse, their longterm prognosis is good.

References

1. Thomson, K. and Turner, D. R. (1976). Mesangial cell cytoplasm and glomerular disease. *J. Pathol.*, **120**, 229–234.

2. Ehrenreich, T. and Churg, J. (1968). Pathology of membranous nephropathy. In Sommers, S. C. (ed.) *Pathology Annual*, Vol. 3, pp. 145–186. (New York: Appleton–Century–Crofts).

3. Habib, R. and Kleinknecht, C. (1975). Membranous nephropathy (extramembranous glomerulonephritis). In Rubin, M. I. and Barratt, T. M. (eds.) *Pediatric Nephrology*, pp. 515–520. (Baltimore: Williams and Wilkins).

4. Evans, D. J. (1974). The pathogenesis of membranous glomerulonephritis, *Lancet*, **1**, 1143–1144.

5. Vernier, R. L., Papermaster, B. W., Olness, K., Binet, E. and Good, R. A. (1960). Morphological studies of the mechanisms of proteinuria. *J. Dis. Child.*, **100**, 476.

6. Munk, F. (1913). Klinische Diagnostik der degenerativen Nierenerkrankungen. *Z. Klin. Med.*, **78**, 1–52.

7. Munk, F. (1916). Die Nephrosen. *Med. Klin.*, **12**, 1019, 1047 and 1073.

8. Ngu, J. L., Barratt, T. M. and Soothill, J. F. (1970). Immunoconglutinin and complement changes in steroid sensitive relapsing nephrotic syndrome of children. *Clin. Exp. Immunol.*, **6**, 109–116.

9. Lagrue, G., Xheneumont, S., Branellec, A., Hirebec, G. and Weil, B. (1975). A vascular permeability factor elaborated from lymphocytes. I. Demonstration in patients with nephrotic syndrome. *Biomed. Express*, **23**, 37–40.

10. Barratt, T. M. and Soothill, J. F. (1970). Control trial of cyclophosphamide in steroid sensitive relapsing nephrotic syndrome of childhood. *Lancet*, **2**, 479–482.

The glomerular lesions so far considered have been diffuse, i.e. they involve all glomeruli. Abnormalities which involve only a proportion of glomeruli are described as 'focal', and where they affect only part of the glomerular tuft, as 'segmental'.

The term 'focal glomerulonephritis' has been applied to proliferative lesions of endocapillary/extracapillary cells, involving some, but not all, glomeruli and usually in a segmental fashion. Focal scarring and fibrinoid necrosis of glomerular tuft are often additional features. A separate category of focal lesions includes those in which segmental or global sclerosis without cellular proliferation affect a proportion of glomeruli (focal segmental/global glomerulosclerosis).

Focal Segmental Proliferative Glomerulonephritis

This diagnosis is applied when proliferative changes affect some glomeruli whilst appearing to spare others. The lesions are generally segmentally distributed, and proliferation of mesangial and/or endothelial cells partially or wholly obliterates a lobule of the glomerular tuft. The more severe segmental lesions commonly show local necrosis and fibrin exudation (Figure 12.1), and this often leads to the formation of adhesions between the affected segment of the tuft and Bowman's capsule (Figure 12.2). Such adhesions commonly elicit local reactive proliferation of adjacent epithelial cells

(Figure 12.3). These may be described as capsular crescents but a clear distinction must be drawn between these small segmental aggregates of epithelial cells, and the prominent proliferation of epithelial cells filling the urinary space in nearly all glomeruli which is the hallmark of diffuse crescentic glomerulonephritis, since the latter has much worse prognostic implications.

The term focal proliferative glomerulonephritis is in most cases inaccurate. Careful examination, particularly using serial sections, usually demonstrates that all, or at least the majority, of glomeruli show some abnormality indicating diffuse rather than focal disease. In the majority of cases an underlying mesangial proliferative type of glomerulonephritis is clearly apparent and the segmental lesions merely represent local accentuation of the changes. This is usually confirmed by the immunochemical techniques which show a diffuse pattern of staining for immunoglobulin and C3 in the mesangium.

Focal segmental proliferative glomerulonephritis is seen in a number of clinical settings including Goodpasture's syndrome, benign recurrent haematuria, infective endocarditis and shunt nephritis. It is also seen when the kidneys are involved in systemic diseases, such as Henoch–Schönlein purpura, lupus erythematosus and polyarteritis nodosa (with or without Wegener's granulomatosis). Distinguishing between these various causes obviously depends heavily on the clinical findings, but additional help is provided by immunochemical analysis (see Table 12.1 and Figures 12.4 and 12.5).

Table 12.1   Immunochemical findings in focal segmental proliferative glomerulonephritis

	Immunofluorescence	Distribution
Recurrent haematuria syndrome	IgA + +, IgG, C3	Mainly mesangial
Goodpasture's syndrome	IgG, (C3)	Linear (GBM)
Infective endocarditis and 'shunt' nephritis	IgG, IgM, C3	Mesangial and capillary loops
Henoch–Schönlein nephritis	IgA, IgG, IgM, C3, fibrin	Mainly mesangial
Lupus nephritis	IgA, IgG, IgM, C3, C1, C4, fibrin	Variable: mesangial and capillary loops
Polyarteritis nodosa and Wegener's granulomatosis	Fibrin only	Focally in tufts and in 'crescents'

Goodpasture's Syndrome

This rare condition is characterized by an association of glomerulonephritis with lung haemorrhage. It is of particular interest as a human example of antiglomerular basement membrane disease. Antibodies against glomerular basement membrane can be demonstrated in the serum, particularly after

bilateral nephrectomy. When eluted from the kidneys of patients with active disease, they are capable of inducing glomerulonephritis when injected into experimental animals[1]. Immunochemical techniques demonstrate the antiglomerular basement membrane antibody as diffuse linear staining of IgG and sometimes C3 along the glomerular capillary basement membranes (Figure 12.6). In the early stages

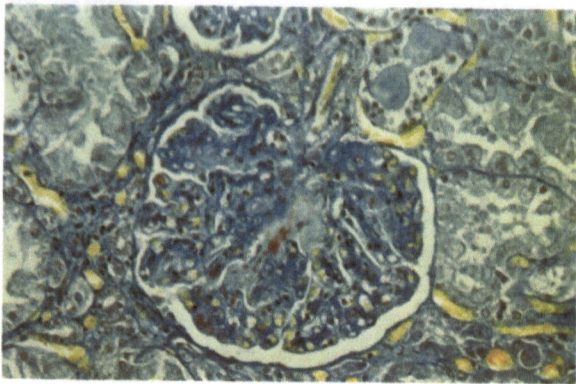

Figure 12.1 Henoch–Schönlein nephritis. In this biopsy proliferative changes affected some glomeruli globally and some segmentally. In the glomerulus illustrated there is a segment of fibrinoid necrosis situated centrally. MSB   × 480.

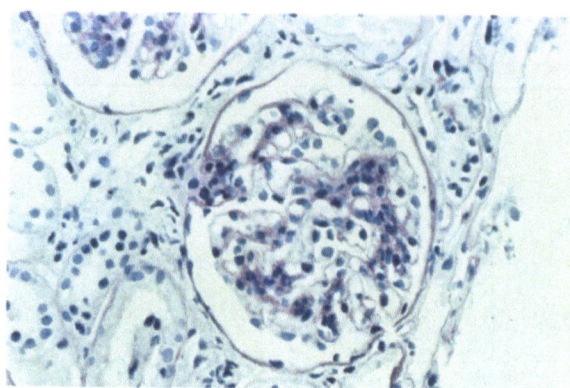

Figure 12.2 Henoch–Schönlein nephritis. The glomerulus shows mild mesangial hypercellularity and a capsular adhesion. PAS   × 480.

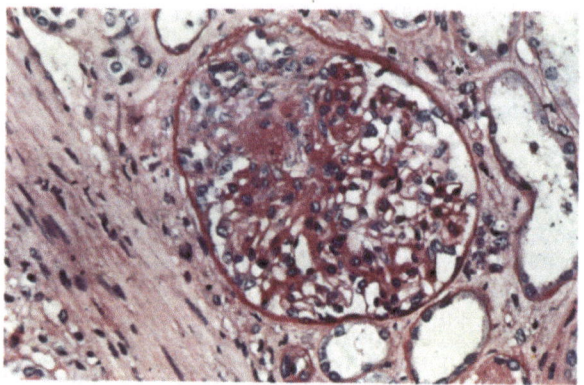

Figure 12.3 Nephritis complicating infective endocarditis. In this glomerulus a segmental lesion in the tuft is associated with conspicuous local reactive proliferation of epithelial cells (capsular 'crescent'). PAS   × 480.

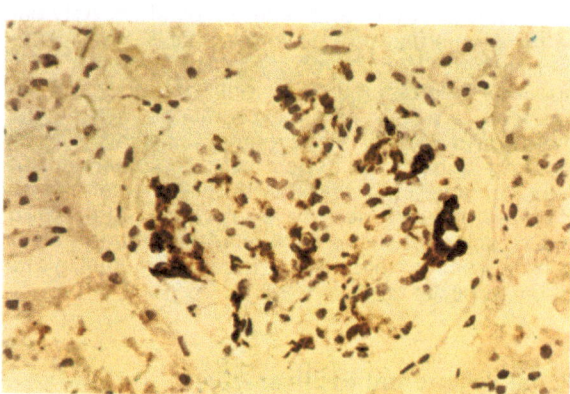

Figure 12.4 Mesangial deposition of IgA in a child with recurrent haematuria. Some IgG and C3 with a similar distribution were also demonstrable. Light microscopy showed a mesangial proliferative glomerulonephritis with focal segmental proliferation. Immunoperoxidase   × 480.

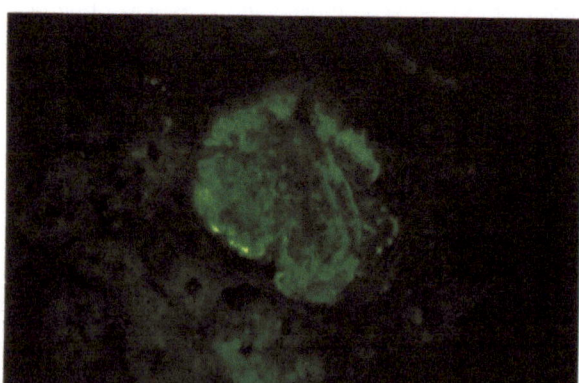

Figure 12.5 Mesangial and peripheral deposition of IgA in Henoch–Schönlein nephritis. Light microscopy showed a focal segmental proliferative glomerulonephritis. Immunofluorescence   × 240.

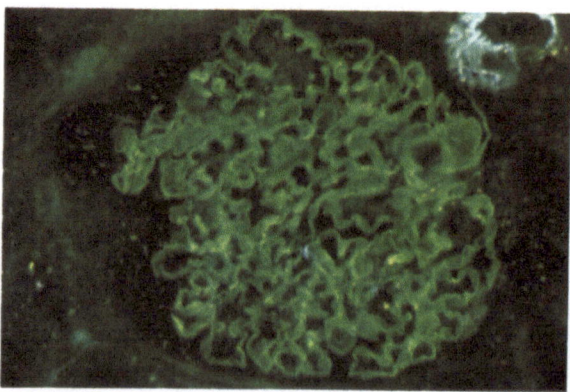

Figure 12.6 Goodpasture's syndrome. Diffuse linear fluorescence with anti-IgG outlining the tuft capillary basement membrane. Immunofluorescence   × 840.

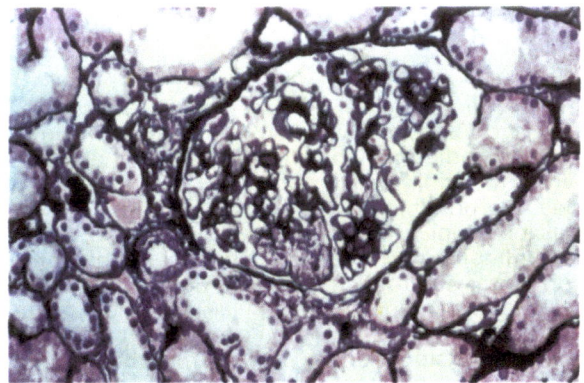

Figure 12.7 Lupus nephritis. A circumscribed area of segmental tuft proliferation and necrosis. Methenamine silver/H & E ×360.

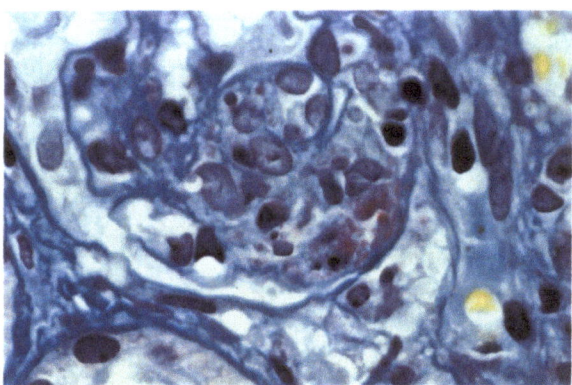

Figure 12.8 Lupus nephritis. Detail of the same segmental lesion in the glomerulus depicted in Figure 12.7. Fibrinoid necrosis and local cellular proliferation in the tuft are apparent. MSB ×1540.

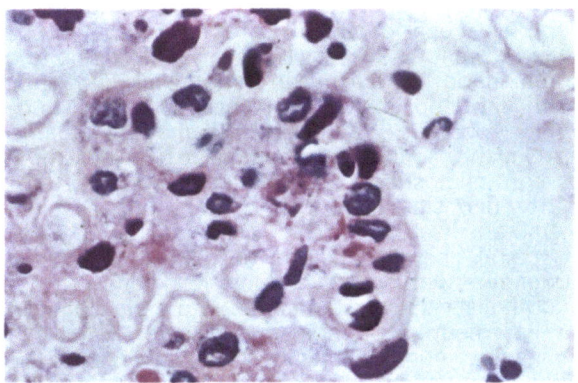

Figure 12.9 Lupus nephritis. A segmental lesion in a glomerular tuft containing haematoxyphil bodies. These are amorphous violaceous aggregates which are smaller than the surrounding nuclei. H & E ×1540.

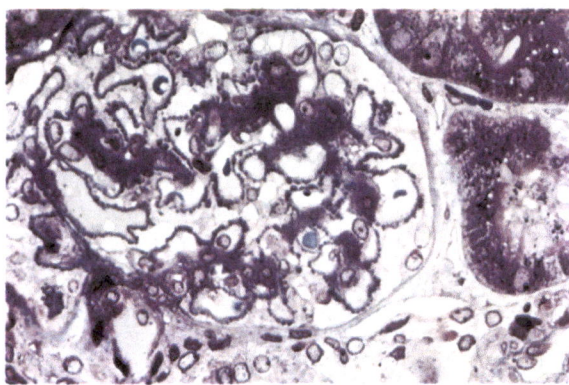

Figure 12.10 Lupus nephritis. A thin 1 μm plastic-embedded section of a glomerulus with extensive membranous transformation and mild mesangial proliferation. Darkly staining deposits are present both on the epithelial aspect of the glomerular capillary basement membrane and within the mesangium. In such cases distinction from idiopathic diffuse membranous glomerulonephritis may be difficult on purely morphological grounds. ×600.

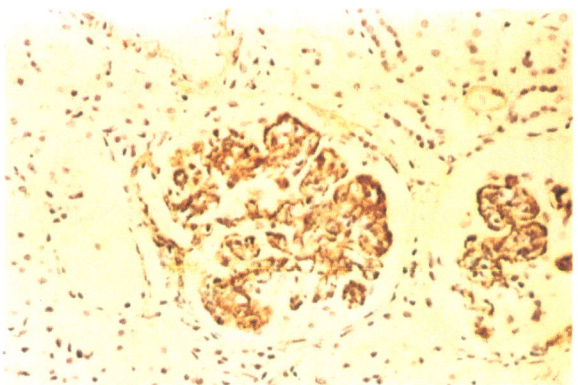

Figure 12.11 Mesangial and peripheral deposition of C1q in lupus nephritis. Paraffin section stained by immunoperoxidase technique. ×240.

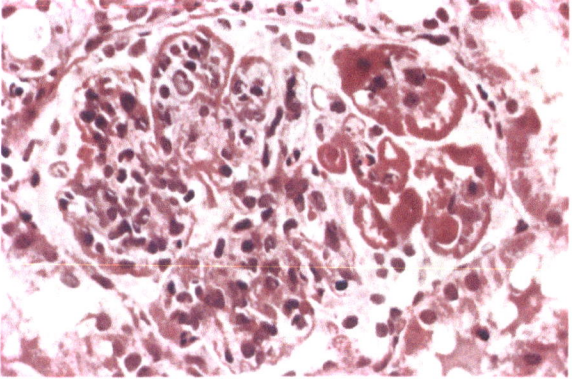

Figure 12.12 Lupus nephritis. A glomerulus showing 'wire looping' of a segment of the tuft, the rest of which shows marked endocapillary proliferative change. H & E ×600.

the glomerulonephritis has a focal segmental pattern, but it usually progresses to a diffuse crescentic type. The prognosis is poor although some therapeutic success has followed removal of circulating antiglomerular basement membrane antibodies by plasmaphoresis prior to transplantation.

Recurrent Haematuria with IgA Deposition

This association has been discussed under mesangial proliferative glomerulonephritis when it was noted that focal segmental accentuation of the glomerular lesions is frequently seen[2] (see page 46).

Infective Endocarditis and Shunt Nephritis

The glomerulonephritis which may complicate infective endocarditis was originally regarded as due to infected microemboli carried from the heart valves. It is now considered to be a form of immune complex disease as indicated by the diffuse granular glomerular deposition of IgG, IgM and C3, and by the report of glomerulonephritis in a case where the tricuspid valve alone was infected[3]. Histologically, focal segmental proliferative glomerulonephritis is the usual pattern, but both diffuse mesangial proliferative and mesangiocapillary lesions may occur.

Shunt nephritis is an occasional complication of patients, usually children, with hydrocephalus treated by ventriculo-atrial shunt. Infection of the shunt, generally by *Staphylococcus albus*, may give rise to an immune complex type of glomerulonephritis. Histologically this resembles the glomerulonephritis complicating infective endocarditis, although the mesangiocapillary pattern is the most common in these patients.

Henoch–Schönlein Nephritis

The Henoch–Schönlein syndrome (anaphylactoid purpura) usually affects children and is characterized by a typical skin rash often accompanied by arthragia and abdominal pain. Renal involvement, indicated by proteinuria and frank or microscopical haematuria, is a fairly common complication, but progressive renal disease is unusual, unless the patient has had recurrent attacks of purpura. The basic histological reaction is a diffuse mesangial proliferative glomerulonephritis, but focal segmental accentuation with small reactive capsular crescents, scarring and capsular adhesion formation are not uncommon even in mild cases. Clinical and histological resolution are the rule, although some residual focal glomerular scarring may be noted in follow-up biopsies. Progressive disease leading to renal failure and hypertension is rare, but crescentic glomerulonephritis with rapid clinical deterioration may occasionally occur.

Lupus Nephritis

Renal involvement in systemic lupus erythematosus is a common and serious complication. Lupus nephritis is often progressive and renal failure is a frequent cause of death in this condition. Histologically a number of patterns of glomerular disease are encountered and their variability, even in a single biopsy specimen, is a useful pointer to the diagnosis. The most frequent change is a focal segmental proliferative glomerulonephritis, superimposed on a mesangial proliferative pattern. Fibrinoid necrosis

within the segmental lesions may occur (Figures 12.7 and 12.8), and very rarely diagnostic 'haematoxyphil bodies' may be encountered (Figure 12.9). When the proliferative reaction is more intense it may be possible to identify a double contour/mesangiocapillary pattern either focally or diffusely. Not infrequently there is membranous transformation with argyrophilic 'spikes' on the epithelial aspects of the glomerular capillary basement membranes (Figure 12.10). Sometimes diffuse membranous transformation occurs and may then present difficulties in differentiation from idiopathic membranous glomerulonephritis. The mesangial cell proliferation which generally accompanies membranous transformation in lupus nephritis is helpful in making this distinction. A wide variety of immunoglobulins (IgA, IgG and IgM), complement fractions (C3, C1q and C4) (Figure 12.11) and fibrin can usually be demonstrated by immunochemical methods in lupus nephritis, and in addition some degree of mesangial cell proliferation is usually present. Both factors help in identifying lupus nephritis. Focal capillary wall thickening (the so-called 'wire loop' lesion) (Figure 12.12) is due to a combination of large sub-endothelial and sub-epithelial deposits which are best seen ultrastructurally (Figure 12.13). The former may be so large as to fill the capillary lumen and have been described by light microscopy as 'hyaline thrombi'. Electron-dense deposits also occur within the basement membrane itself and in the mesangium. Other ultrastructural changes include collections of tubular structures within the endoplasmic reticulum of endothelial cells, and structures within the glomerular basement membrane composed of lattices of concentric curves resembling 'fingerprints'. The tubular structures in endothelial cells have been compared with virus particles[4], but are probably products of cell injury and in any case are not peculiar to lupus nephritis. Electron-dense deposits, presumably immune complexes, are also occasionally encountered along tubular basement membranes (Figure 12.14).

Polyarteritis Nodosa

This disorder is characterized by random focal necrotizing inflammation affecting the walls of medium-sized or small arterial vessels throughout the body. Occasionally there is an associated necrotizing and granulomatous inflammation in the lungs and upper respiratory tract (Wegener's granulomatosis). In the kidney there may be involvement of muscular arteries down to arcuate size (the macroscopic form; Figure 12.15) or of small arterioles and capillaries including those of the glomerular tufts (the microscopic form). The latter is the type most frequently encountered in biopsy material. Arteritic lesions of arterioles are only occasionally seen in such specimens (Figures 12.16 and 12.17). The glomerular reaction is a focal segmental proliferation with fibrinoid necrosis of some segments as a prominent feature (Figure 12.18). This often progresses to a diffuse extracapillary glomerulonephritis with prominent capsular crescent formation. Immunochemical techniques fail to demonstrate immunoglobulins or complement but give a strongly postive reaction for fibrin.

Focal Segmental/Global Glomerulosclerosis

For some years it has been recognized that a small proportion of nephrotic children with apparent 'minimal change' disease have a poorer prognosis than is usual in that condition. They tend to develop progressive renal failure, usually slowly over a number of years, but occasionally over a much shorter period. There are a number of clinical features which distinguish these patients from those with classical 'minimal change' disease. They tend to be older with a higher proportion of girls than boys, and their nephrotic syndrome is usually steroid-resistant. They may have microscopic haematuria and may be hypertensive. A proportion of glomeruli show sclerosis which may be segmental or global (i.e. involving the whole glomerular tuft) (Figure 12.19). The segmental lesions are characterized by the presence of hyaline eosinophilic material which can be shown by electron microscopy to be situated in the sub-endothelial position in early lesions[5] (Figure 12.20). Evolution of the lesion results in obliteration and collapse of affected capillary loops and an increase in mesangial matrix without endocapillary proliferation (Figure 12.21). The lesions often start near the hilum of the glomerulus and hyaline deposits may also be found in the adjacent afferent arteriole. The segmental lesions often become adherent to Bowman's capsule and sometimes there are small local reactive aggregates of adjacent epithelial cells (Figure 12.22). The lesions tend to be progressive so that eventually the whole glomerular tuft becomes sclerosed (global sclerosis), and in serial biopsies there is a tendency for more and more glomeruli to be affected. Although the lesion is focal, involvement of glomeruli is not random, particularly early in the process (Figure 12.23). The first glomeruli to be affected are those in the deep juxtamedullary cortex[6]. This non-random distribution of lesions may give rise to difficulties in biopsy diagnosis. If the biopsy contains only superficial cortex, only glomeruli normal to light microscopy may be found and an erroneous diagnosis of 'minimal change' disease made. Even when the biopsy samples the deep cortex, lesions may be very sparse early in the disease. Their demonstration may require a very careful hunt in serial sections of the biopsy specimen, which may be indicated if clinical data such as non-response to steroids make a diagnosis of minimal change disease less likely (Figure 12.24). Tubules associated with the sclerosed glomeruli become atrophic, and the presence of atrophic tubules, particularly in a child's biopsy, should alert the observer. Even if typical glomerular lesions are not apparent in the initial sections, further serial sections may reveal them.

Immunofluorescence microscopy is usually negative, but sometimes immunoglobulins (particularly IgM) and C3 may be seen and a useful diagnostic point is that they are deposited only in the sclerotic lesions. Occasionally, completely sclerosed glomeruli are seen in renal biopsy specimens with little else of note to be seen, and this may lead to difficulties in interpretation.

In young children with the nephrotic syndrome, occasional totally hyalinized glomeruli may represent local developmental defects where nephrons have failed to establish their proper connections with branches of the ureteric bud. These cases may be distinguished by the absence of tubular atrophy or glomeruli showing segmental lesions. Nash et al.[7], have shown that such nephrotic children with only focal global sclerosis have a natural history like that of minimal change disease.

Some children with frequently relapsing steroid-sensitive nephrotic syndrome, whose initial biopsy shows no significant abnormality on light microscopy, may develop lesions of focal segmental glomerulosclerosis after a number of years. They nevertheless have a much better prognosis than patients whose biopsies at presentation show focal glomerulosclerosis.

Occasional segmentally scarred glomeruli may be found under a number of circumstances, such as hypertensive nephrosclerosis, chronic pyelonephritis or following severe diffuse endocapillary or segmental proliferative glomerulonephritis. Evaluation of the clinical as well as the pathological findings are needed for the correct interpretation of these lesions.

Diffuse Global Glomerulosclerosis

Diffuse glomerular scarring accompanied by widespread tubular and interstitial changes and arteriosclerosis occurs with any type of glomerulonephritis as it progresses to chronic renal failure. These changes may mask or obliterate any features which allow a more specific histological diagnosis and for these the category of diffuse global glomerulosclerosis is reserved. Specimens from patients maintained on longterm chronic dialysis not infrequently fall into this group.

References

1. Lerner, R. A., Glassock, R. J. and Dixon, F. J. (1967). The role of antiglomerular basement membrane antibody in the pathogenesis of human glomerulonephritis. *J. Exp. Med.*, **126**, 989–1004.

2. Berger, J., Yaneva, H. and Hinglais, N. (1971). Immunochemistry of glomerulonephritis. In Hamburger, J., Grosnier, J. and Maxwell, M. H. (eds.). *Advances in Nephrology*. Vol. 1, pp. 11–30. (Chicago: Year Book Medical Publishers).

3. Bain, R. C., Edwards, J. E., Schiegley, C. H. and Geruci, J. E. (1958). Right-sided bacterial endocarditis and endarteritis: a clinical and pathological study. *Am. J. Med.*, **24**, 98–110.

4. Andres, G. A., Spiele, H. and McCluskey, R. T. (1972). Virus-like structures in systemic lupus erythematosus. *Prog. Clin. Immunol.*, **1**, 23–44.

5. Churg, J. and Grishman, E. (1973). Nephrotic syndrome of focal glomerular sclerosis. In Becker, E. L. (ed.) *Cornell Seminars in Nephrology*, pp. 34–43. (New York: John Wiley).

6. Rich, A. R. (1957). A hitherto undescribed vulnerability of the juxtamedullary glomeruli in lipid nephrosis. *Bull. Johns Hopkins Hosp.*, **100**, 173–186.

7. Nash, M. A., Greiger, I., Olbing, H., Bernstein, J., Bennett, B. and Spitzer, A. The significance of focal sclerotic lesions of glomeruli in children. *J. Paediatr.*, **88**, 806–813.

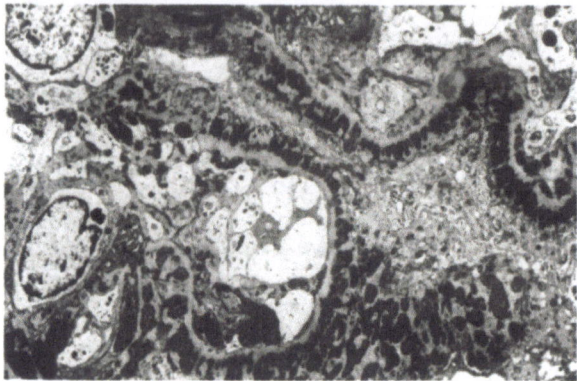

Figure 12.13 Ultrastructural appearance of the 'wire loop' lesion illustrated in Figure 12.12. There are numerous large deposits on both sides of the glomerular capillary basement membrane.   ×3200.

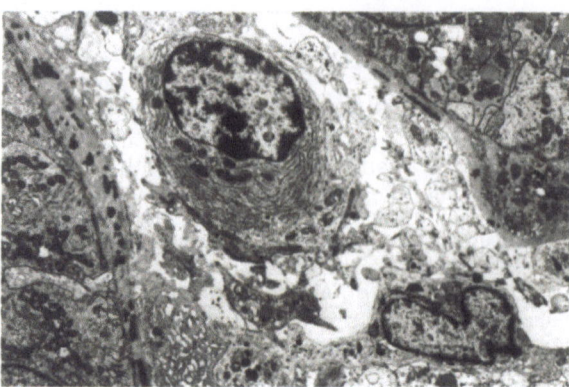

Figure 12.14 Lupus nephritis. Ultrastructural appearance of electron-dense deposits within the basement membranes of adjacent tubules (separated by an intervening plasma cell in the interstitium).   ×4100.

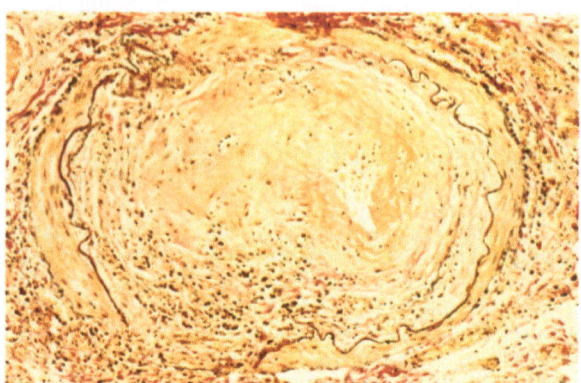

Figure 12.15 'Healed' polyarteritis nodosa in an arcuate artery. There is fibrous thickening of the intima extending into the media and adventitia. The internal elastic lamina is interrupted in the region of the fibrous scarring indicating previous necrosis of the wall. Elastic/van Gieson   ×240.

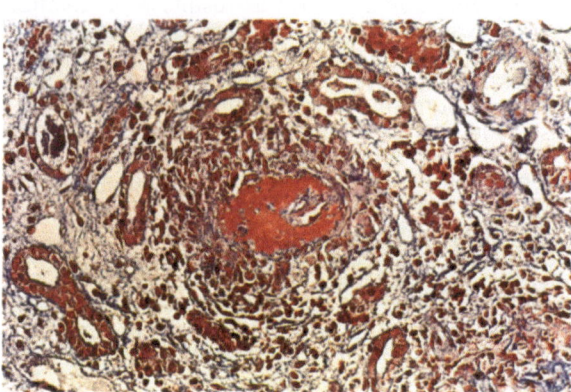

Figure 12.16 Fibrinoid necrosis and active chronic inflammation of an arteriole in polyarteritis nodosa. MSB   ×480.

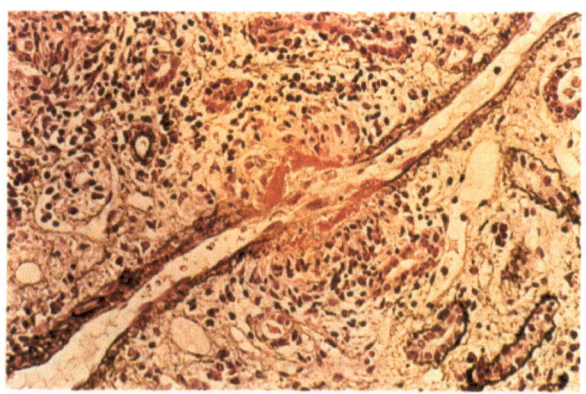

Figure 12.17 Arteritic lesion of polyarteritis nodosa affecting a small interlobular artery which has been sectioned longitudinally and illustrates the focal nature of the disease. Methenamine silver/H & E   ×480.

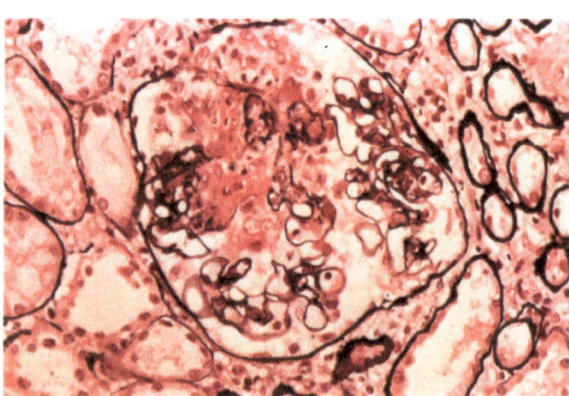

Figure 12.18 Polyarteritis nodosa. A segmental area of tuft necrosis with both endocapillary and extracapillary cellular proliferation. Methenamine silver   ×600.

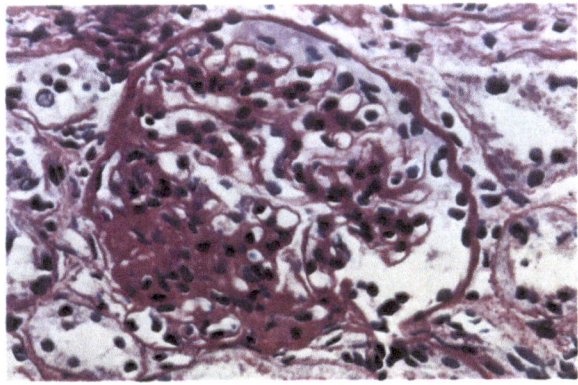

Figure 12.19 Focal glomerulosclerosis. A glomerulus showing segmental sclerosis involving nearly half of the tuft. Other glomeruli in this biopsy from a 7-year-old girl with the nephrotic syndrome were either normal to light microscopy or globally sclerosed. Areas of tubular atrophy associated with the abnormal glomeruli were present. PAS × 600.

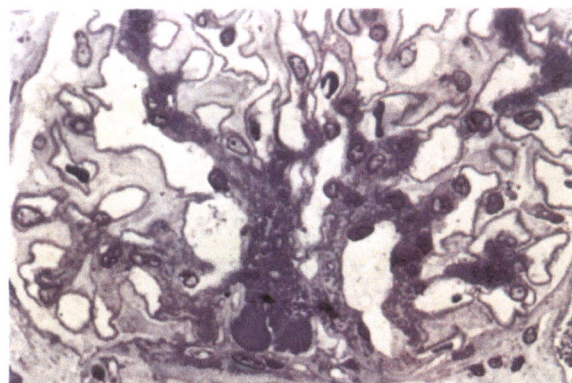

Figure 12.20 Focal glomerulosclerosis. Part of the glomerular tuft showing hyaline sub-endothelial deposits adjacent to the hilum. Plastic-embedded section. Toluidine blue × 1200.

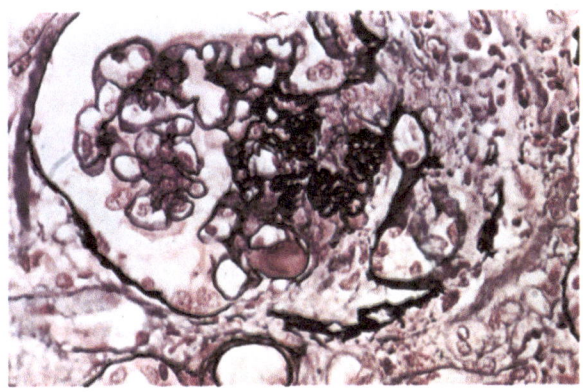

Figure 12.21 Focal glomerulosclerosis. A glomerulus showing segmental sclerosis and collapse with a prominent sub-endothelial deposit almost obliterating one capillary loop. Methenamine silver/H & E × 720.

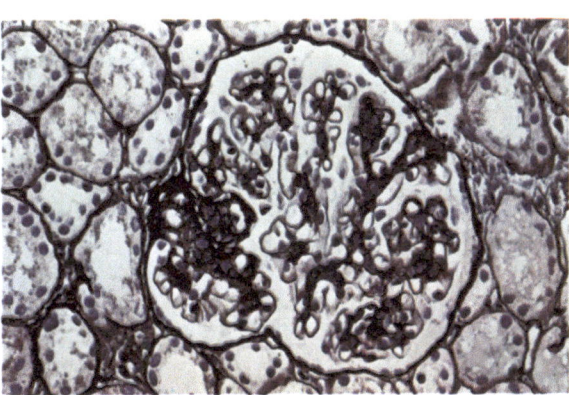

Figure 12.22 Focal glomerulosclerosis. A glomerulus showing two localized areas of tuft sclerosis each associated with capsular adhesions. Methenamine silver/H & E × 600.

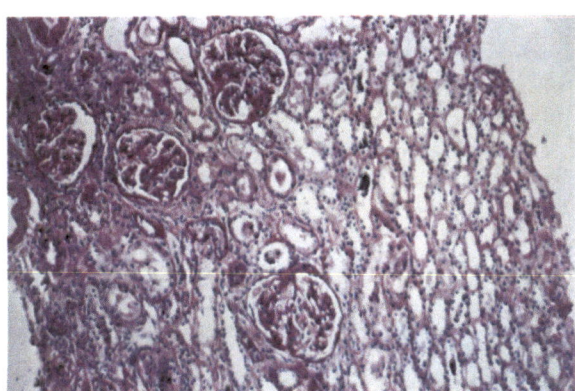

Figure 12.23 Focal glomerulosclerosis. Four glomeruli from the juxtamedullary cortex showing segmental lesions, and atrophy of associated tubules. Other more superficial glomeruli in this biopsy from an 8-year-old boy with the nephrotic syndrome were normal to light microscopy. PAS × 160.

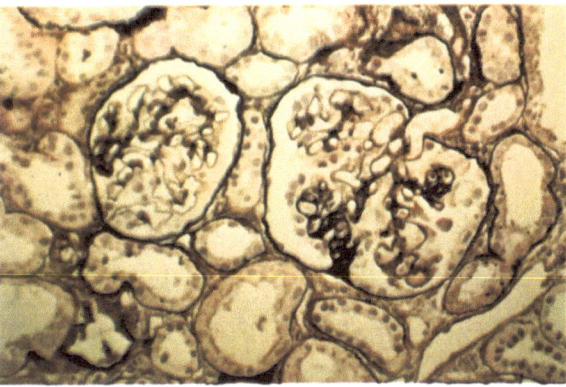

Figure 12.24 Focal glomerulosclerosis. Two glomeruli showing focal segmental tuft sclerosis in a child with steroid-resistant nephrotic syndrome. Initial sections showed no glomerular lesions by light microscopy, although there were foci of tubular atrophy. The glomerular lesions were discovered only after serial sectioning of the biopsy. Methenamine silver × 360.

Microangiopathic Haemolytic Anaemia and Scleroderma

Renal damage may result from glomerular fibrin deposition. This occurs in some forms of glomerulonephritis and can cause, for example, capsular crescent formation (Figures 13.1 and 13.2) and local scarring in some segmental proliferative lesions. Deposition of fibrin may be precipitated by antigen–antibody complexes which are capable of releasing thrombogenic substances from platelets, and this probably explains its association with immunologically-mediated diseases such as glomerulonephritis. However, intravascular coagulation induced by other non-immunological mechanisms may also result in glomerular fibrin deposition. The associated changes in the glomeruli have been elegantly demonstrated in rabbits by Vassalli et al.[1] and include endocapillary cell proliferation, capsular crescent formation, leukocyte infiltration, deposition of fibrin and its derivatives (seen ultrastructurally as deposits of varying electron density) in the mesangium and the widened sub-endothelial space, and swelling of endothelial cells. These changes may progress to glomerular hyalinization with increased amounts of mesangial matrix, and there may be focal reduplication of the lamina densa seen in methenamine silver preparations. Similar changes have been described by Kincaid-Smith[2] in renal biopsy specimens from patients with intravascular coagulation, and it has been claimed that the changes may be prevented by anticoagulant therapy[3].

Microangiopathic Haemolytic Anaemia

This is a form of haemolytic anaemia associated with fragmented and deformed red cells ('burr cells') in the blood, and fibrin deposition in small vessels including glomerular capillaries. Thrombocytopenia is usually an additional feature, and direct Coombs' testing is generally negative. It is suggested[4] that the destruction of red cells is mechanical and results from trauma and distortion following contact with the damaged endothelium and fibrin thrombi in small blood vessels; thrombocytopenia is similarly related to contact between platelets and damaged blood vessels, causing their adherence and initiating further intravascular coagulation. Microangiopathic haemolytic anaemia may therefore occur under a number of conditions where disseminated intravascular coagulation occurs.

Haemolytic Uraemic Syndrome

This describes the combination of haemolytic anaemia and thrombocytopenia with renal failure. Children are usually affected; over 90% of cases occur under the age of 4 years and the majority occur in the first year of life. The sexes are affected equally, but there is a seasonal variation, the condition being commoner in the summer and autumn in the northern hemisphere. Very commonly an acute infection, usually of the gastro-intestinal tract, precedes the attack by a few days. The disease is characterized by an acute onset of jaundice, anaemia and thrombocytopenia with deformed and fragmented red cells in the peripheral blood. This is accompanied by acute renal failure and often hypertension; congestive cardiac failure and pulmonary oedema may complicate the picture[5].

Changes in the kidney are variable. Rarely there is massive bilateral renal cortical necrosis. More commonly there is swelling of the glomerular tufts, with global and segmental endocapillary cell proliferation and occasional fibrin and platelet thrombi occluding glomerular tufts, sometimes afferent arterioles or even small arteries (Figures 13.3 and 13.4). Scattered capsular crescents may also be seen. Ultrastructurally, electron-dense material resembling fibrin is deposited in the widened sub-endothelial space and in the mesangium; some glomerular capillary lumina are occluded by mixtures of fibrin, deformed red cells and platelet aggregates. Immunofluorescence microscopy reveals fibrin deposits along capillary loops and in the mesangium, but immunoglobulins are generally absent.

Evolution of the renal lesion can be correlated with the severity of the initial attack. In the minority with prolonged anuria, glomerular scarring is severe, and whole glomeruli and segments of glomeruli become completely solidified and acellular. Interstitial fibrosis and tubular atrophy are marked and haemosiderin deposition (reflecting haemoglobulinuria occurring in the acute phase) is conspicuous (Figure 13.5). Small arteries and arterioles show considerable intimal hyperplasia and luminal narrowing.

Scleroderma (Progressive Systemic Sclerosis)

This condition is characterized by inflammatory and fibrotic changes throughout the interstitium of many organs, but principally affects the skin. It is usually regarded as an immunological disorder and is classified as a 'connective tissue' disease like rheumatoid arthritis, systemic lupus erythematosus and Sjögren's syndrome, with which it has certain similarities and overlapping features both clinically and morphologically. Scleroderma affects women twice as commonly as men, and usually presents between the third and fifth decades. The kidneys are frequently affected and renal failure was the cause of death in nearly half the cases in one large series[6]. Clinically, renal failure can sometimes develop rapidly and may

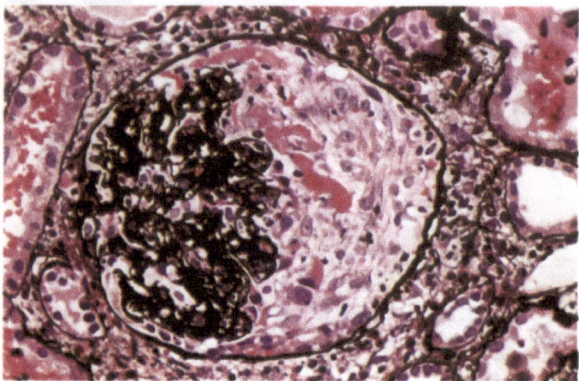

Figure 13.1 Disseminated intravascular coagulation (DIC). Marked extracapillary cellular proliferation (capsular crescent formation) with fibrin deposition. The underlying tuft is collapsed. H & E/Methenamine silver × 600.

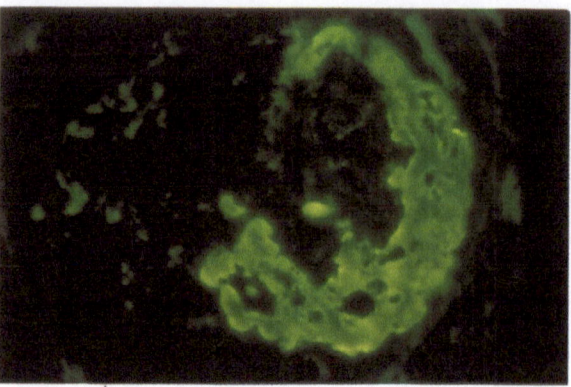

Figure 13.2 DIC. Immunofluorescence microscopy in the same case illustrated in Figure 13.1, showing fibrin deposition within the capsular crescent. × 600.

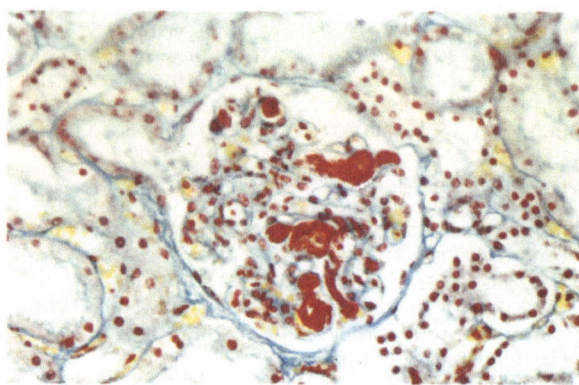

Figure 13.3 DIC/haemolytic–uraemic syndrome. In the acute stage the changes are as in this case where fibrin thrombi occlude several capillary loops within the glomerular tuft. MSB × 480.

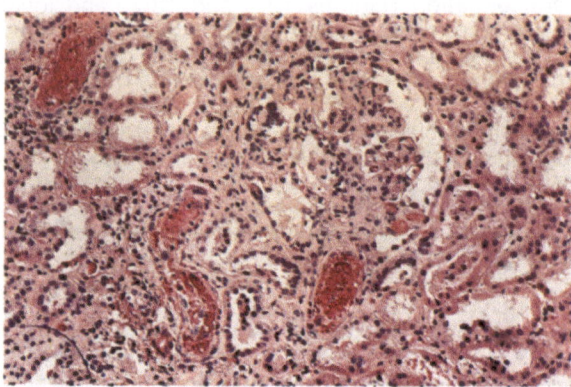

Figure 13.4 DIC/haemolytic–uraemic syndrome. An area of renal cortex showing segmental endocapillary proliferation in a capillary tuft, associated with micro-thrombus formation within the tuft, in the afferent arteriole and in an adjacent small interlobular artery. The glomerular tuft also shows capsular adhesions with mild reactive change in the adjacent epithelial cell. H & E × 240.

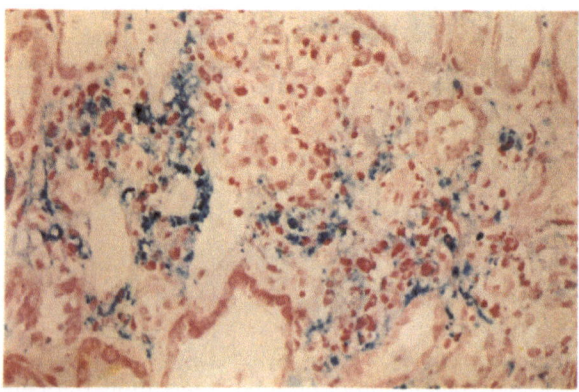

Figure 13.5 DIC/haemolytic–uraemic syndrome. Marked deposition of stainable iron in tubular epithelium and renal interstitium, reflecting extensive haemolysis. Perl's iron × 600.

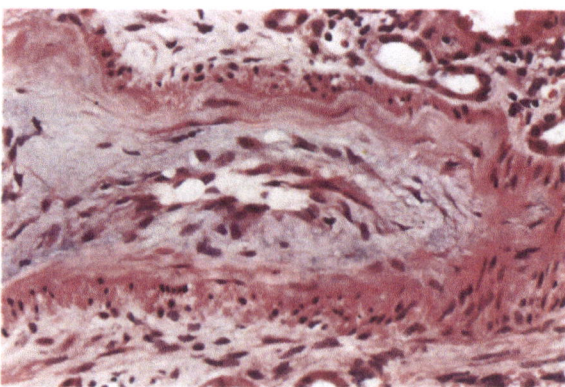

Figure 13.6 Scleroderma. An interlobular artery showing loose mucinous intimal thickening causing luminal narrowing. H & E × 600.

be accompanied by accelerated hypertension. The pathological changes in the kidneys in such cases have a number of features in common with those seen in intravascular coagulation and Kincaid-Smith[2] includes acute scleroderma amongst the list of conditions in which coagulation plays a part. Grossly the kidneys are normal or slightly increased in size. Petechial haemorrhages may be apparent on the subcapsular surfaces and multiple small infarcts may be present. Microscopically the glomeruli show a variety of changes. Some appear normal whilst others show acellular hyalinization of the tufts. Some show fibrin thrombi or areas of fibrinoid necrosis which may be in continuity with similar changes in afferent arterioles. Interlobular arteries show a characteristic mucinous or loose collagenous intimal thickening, often with considerable luminal narrowing (Figure 13.6). Larger arteries of arcuate or interlobar size are often normal. There is widespread tubular atrophy and interstitial fibrosis, and areas of infarction may be seen. Immunofluorescence microscopy demonstrates fibrin deposition in glomeruli, arterioles and affected interlobular arteries. Ultrastructurally, sub-endothelial and mesangial hyaline deposits in glomeruli and fibrinoid intimal deposits in interlobular arteries have been reported[7].

References

1. Vassalli, P., Simon, G. and Rouiller, C. (1963). Electron microscopic study of glomerular lesions resulting from intravascular fibrin formation. *Am. J. Pathol.*, **43**, 578–617.

2. Kincaid-Smith, P. (1973). The role of coagulation in obliteration of glomerular capillaries. In Kincaid-Smith, P., Mathew, T. H. and Becker, E. L. (eds.) *Glomerulonephritis; Morphology, Natural History and Treatment*, p. 871. (New York: Wiley).

3. Kincaid-Smith, P., Laver, M. C. and Fairley, K. F. (1970). Dipyridamole and anticoagulants in renal disease due to glomerular and vascular lesions: a new approach to therapy. *Med. J. Aust.*, **1**, 145–151.

4. Brain, M. C., Dacie, J. V. and Hourihane, D. O'B. (1962). Microangiopathic haemolytic anaemia: The possible role of vascular lesions in pathogenesis. *Br. J. Haematol.*, **8**, 358–374.

5. Lieberman, E., Heuser, E., Donnell, G. N., Landing, B. H. and Hammond, G. D. (1966). Hemolytic–uremic syndrome. Clinical and pathological considerations. *N. Engl. J. Med.*, **275**, 227–236.

6. Rodnan, G. P. (1963). The natural history of progressive systemic sclerosis (diffuse scleroderma). *Bull. Rheum. Dis.*, **13**, 301–304.

7. Vidt, D. G., Robertson, A. L. Jr. and Deodhar, S. D. (1971). Renal changes in progressive systemic sclerosis. Report of five cases. *Cleveland Clin. Quart.*, **38**, 141–146.

The authors are grateful to Dr M. K. MacDonald for providing Figure 13.4.

Renal Infections

Urinary tract infections are relatively common during pregnancy and the puerperium, and sometimes the upper urinary tract and kidney are involved. Quite often urinary infection is asymptomatic and only discovered on routine urine culture. Discovery of urinary infection, whether overt or covert, is important since treatment lessens the risk of pyelonephritis which in pregnancy is usually acute and generally occurs after the 20th week. The risk is probably related to the physiological dilatation and reduced peristalsis of the ureter and renal pelvis which occurs during pregnancy and often persists for some weeks after delivery[1]. The ureteric dilatation, formerly thought to be due to compression of the ureter at the pelvic brim by the gravid uterus, is probably an hormonal effect.

Toxaemia of Pregnancy

This rather unsatisfactory term denotes the development of proteinuria, oedema and hypertension during pregnancy. This may occur in previously normal women, usually in the later stages of pregnancy (36 weeks or more) when the condition is referred to as pre-eclampsia. Patients with essential hypertension or chronic renal disease such as glomerulonephritis may also show a rise in blood pressure accompanied by oedema and proteinuria, and in these women it often occurs at an earlier stage of pregnancy. Pre-eclampsia may progress to eclampsia which is a serious and possibly life-threatening condition characterized by epileptiform fits and usually accompanied by a sharp rise in blood pressure to high levels.

Patients with pre-eclampsia/eclampsia show characteristic changes on renal biopsy, the severity of which parallels their clinical condition.

By light microscopy all the glomeruli are enlarged; the tufts show exaggerated lobulation and fill the urinary spaces. Capillary lumina are reduced so that the glomeruli appear abnormally solid, although there is little or no increased cellularity. This appearance is due to endothelial cell and, to a lesser extent, mesangial cell swelling. The capillary walls are thickened, but this is due to endothelial swelling rather than basement membrane thickening as is well demonstrated in Alcian blue/PAS preparations. Epithelial cells are also swollen and may exhibit cytoplasmic hyaline droplets. Tubules show little alteration beyond hyaline droplet change; abnormalities of the interstitium and blood vessels are also inconspicuous (Figures 14.1, 14.2 and 14.3). Arteries may show endothelial swelling and occasionally hyaline thickening of their walls.

Electron microscopy confirms the endothelial and mesangial cell swelling which is associated with cytoplasmic vacuolation and droplet formation. Basement membrane changes are seen only in severe cases when there may be localized homogeneous thickening or occasionally 'reduplication' with mesangial interposition to give a double contour effect which may also be seen by light microscopy in silver methenamine preparations (Figures 14.5 and 14.6). Kincaid-Smith[2] has described electron-lucent zones in the sub-endothelium in pre-eclampsia, a change which is a feature common to conditions associated with fibrin deposition (Figures 14.7 and 14.8). Electron-dense, finely granular or fibrillary material may be seen in endothelial cell cytoplasm, in the sub-endothelium, or apparently in the capillary lumen adjoining endothelial cells (Figure 14.9). Whilst this material lacks the periodicity of fibrin, it is regarded by McKay[3] as a type of precipitated fibrinogen and has been described by other authors as fibrinoid. This is supported by the findings on immunofluorescence microscopy which show positive fluorescence along capillary loops and in the mesangium with antisera against fibrinogen, but usually negative results with antisera to immunoglobulins.

These morphological findings together with coagulation studies strongly support the concept that intravascular coagulation is involved in the pathogenesis of the renal lesion in pre-eclampsia/eclampsia. Lesions in the liver, brain, lung and adrenal which may be found at autopsy in patients dying of eclampsia may also be explained on this basis, although the triggering mechanism initiating intravascular coagulation remains obscure.

Clinical improvement, even in severe cases, is usually dramatic within a short time of delivery. In general this is accompanied by complete resolution of the renal lesion. Minor residual changes have occasionally been described, particularly focal capillary wall thickening and basement membrane 'reduplication' although even this type of lesion may resolve.

Acute Postpartum Renal Failure

A rare complication of the first few weeks of the postpartum period is the development of acute renal failure, which may be complicated by a haemolytic anaemia and thrombocytopenia and for this reason is sometimes grouped with the haemolytic–uraemic syndrome. The renal pathology closely resembles that described in scleroderma, and Kincaid-Smith[2] has described ultrastructural changes in the glomeruli such as electron-lucent zones in the sub-

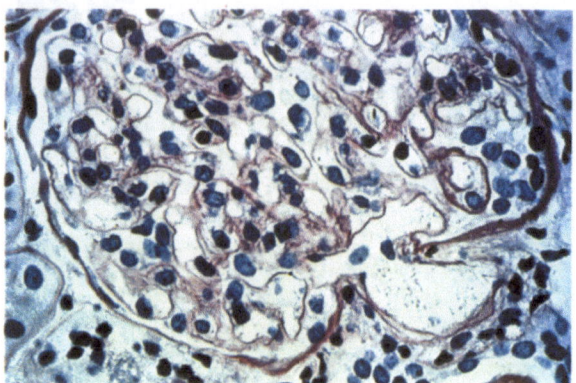

Figure 14.1 Pre-eclampsia. In their mildest form, the glomerular changes are characterized by some swelling of endothelial and mesangial cell cytoplasm. PAS × 960.

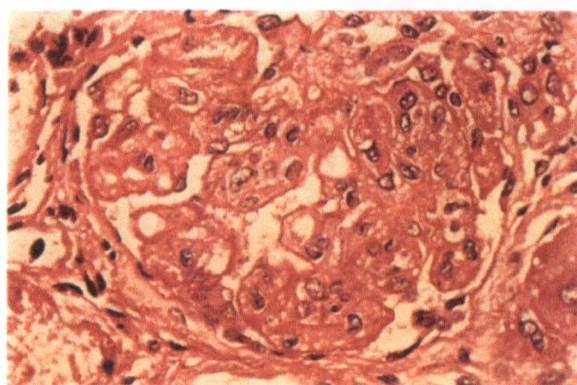

Figure 14.2 Pre-eclampsia. A case showing more marked glomerular changes. Endothelial and mesangial cell swelling has caused accentuated lobulation and enlargement of the glomerular tuft which virtually fills the urinary space. In addition, capillary lumina within the glomerular tuft are reduced. PAS × 960.

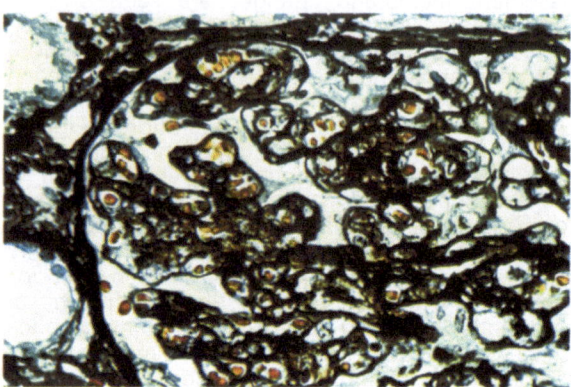

Figure 14.3 Pre-eclampsia. In the fully developed glomerular lesion, there is diffuse mesangial increase and patchy basement membrane reduplication. Methenamine silver × 960.

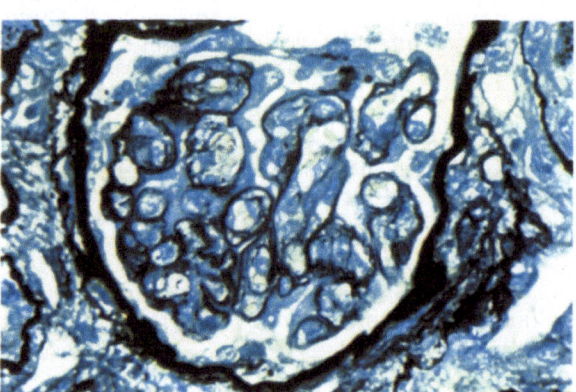

Figure 14.4 Postpartum acute renal failure. A glomerulus showing patchy reduplication of the glomerular basement membrane with mesangial interposition, in a follow-up biopsy. Methenamine silver × 960.

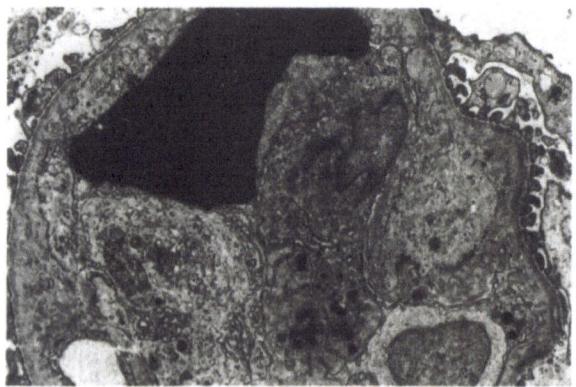

Figure 14.5 Pre-eclampsia. Electron micrograph of a glomerular capillary loop showing endothelial cell swelling, with platelets, a red blood cell and a leukocyte filling the reduced capillary lumen. × 4900.

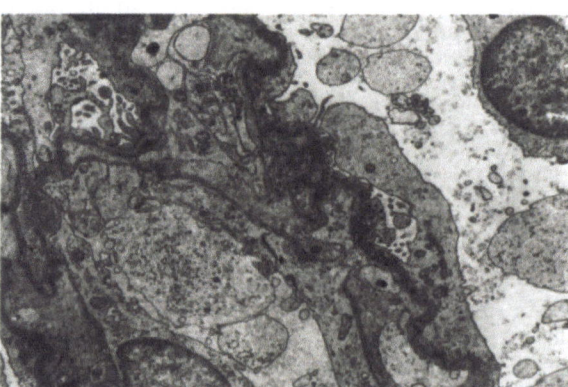

Figure 14.6 Pre-eclampsia. Electron micrograph of a capillary loop, showing endothelial cell swelling and mesangial interposition between the endothelium and the glomerular basement membrane. × 2460.

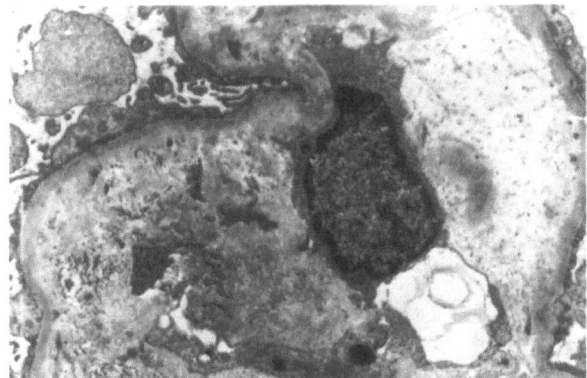

Figure 14.7 Pre-eclampsia. Electron micrograph showing a wide electron lucent zone in the sub-endothelial space, in which fibrillary electron dense material can be seen in some parts. × 4900.

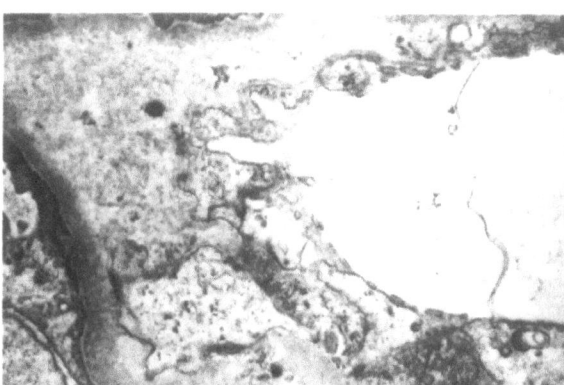

Figure 14.8 Pre-eclampsia. Similar changes to those described in Figure 13.13, showing mesangial cell processes in the sub-endothelial space and adjacent dark fibrillary material. × 12 300.

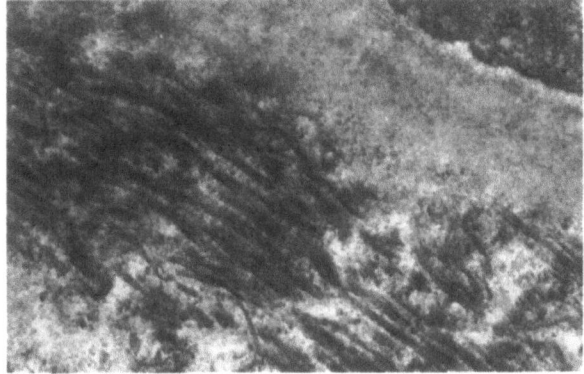

Figure 14.9 Pre-eclampsia. High power electron micrograph of fibrillary material (fibrinoid), in the sub-endothelial space. × 30 300.

endothelium and fibrillary or granular deposits, which she regards as common to those conditions where fibrin deposition is the main pathogenic mechanism. Many patients with this lesion die, although recovery may occur following anti-coagulant therapy. Follow-up renal biopsies in patients who do recover may show focal glomerular basement membrane reduplication with mesangial interposition ('double contours') on methenamine silver staining (Figure 14.4).

Renal Cortical Necrosis

This condition as a complication of pregnancy has already been described.

References

1. Traut, H. F., and McLane, C. M. (1936). Physiological changes in the ureter associated with pregnancy. *Surg. Gynaecol. Obstet.*, **62**, 65–70.

2. Kincaid-Smith, P. (1973). The similarity of lesions and underlying mechanisms in pre-eclamptic toxaemia and post-partum renal failure. Studies in the acute stage and during follow-up. In Kincaid-Smith, P., Mathew, T. H. and Becker, E. L. (eds.) *Glomerulonephritis; Morphology, Natural History, and Treatment*, p. 1013. (New York: Wiley).

3. McKay, D. G. (1964). Clinical significance of the pathology of toxaemia of pregnancy. *Circulation*, **30** (suppl. II), 66–75.

The authors are grateful to Dr M. K. MacDonald for providing Figures 14.1, 14.2, 14.3, 14.4, 14.5, 14.6, 14.7, 14.8 and 14.9.

Amyloidosis and Myelomatosis

15

Amyloidosis

Amyloid is an abnormal, eosinophilic, hyaline proteinaceous material which is deposited in tissues in certain circumstances. Deposition may be localized, but is usually widely distributed throughout the body. Traditionally, generalized amyloidosis is classified as primary or secondary. Primary amyloidosis is either idiopathic or a complication of multiple myelomatosis; secondary amyloidosis follows a number of longstanding chronic inflammatory diseases. In the past, chronic suppurative diseases such as osteomyelitis or bronchiectasis, tertiary syphilis or caseous tuberculosis were the common precursors. At the present time lepromatous leprosy, rheumatoid arthritis, malignant disease (notably Hodgkin's disease and renal carcinoma), decubitus ulceration and suppurative pyelonephritis in patients with longstanding paraplegia are more usual underlying causes.

Amyloid has a number of staining properties by which it can be identified microscopically, including an affinity for Congo red (with a characteristic apple green birefringence when viewed by polarized light), metachromatic staining with methyl violet and fluorescence with ultraviolet light following thioflavin-T treatment.

Under the electron microscope amyloid has a characteristic fibrillary structure, although it is not a single protein. In primary amyloidosis it is composed of immunoglobulin light chains (or parts of them). In secondary amyloidosis (amyloid AA) it has a different amino acid sequence and the fibrils are formed from different polypeptide fragments derived from immunoglobulins or some other source[1].

Renal amyloid deposition is common in both primary and secondary amyloidosis, and in the rare familial forms (particularly familial Mediterranean fever). Clinically, renal involvement is indicated by proteinuria which is often heavy and may result in the nephrotic syndrome. When extensive, renal amyloidosis causes renal failure which may be accompanied by hypertension. Renal tubular acidosis and hyperkalaemia also occur occasionally.

The kidneys are usually enlarged (although occasionally reduced in size), pale in colour and firm in consistency. Extensive amyloid deposition can be demonstrated macroscopically by the application of a solution of iodine in dilute sulphuric acid to the cut surface of the gross specimen when the amyloid stains a mahogany brown colour (Figure 15.1).

Microscopically, amyloid can usually be identified in the glomeruli even in the earliest stages, although they may be spared in some cases of amyloidosis complicating myelomatosis. Early glomerular deposits form between capillary basement membranes and the mesangium as small eosinophilic nodules (Figures 15.2, 15.3 and 15.4). These may be inconspicuous unless specifically sought and are occasionally only identified in the electron microscope. Occasionally, too, amyloid may be deposited in a spicular fashion along the epithelial aspect of the glomerular basement membrane (Figures 15.12, 15.13 and 15.14) to give an appearance in methenamine silver preparations which could be mistaken for focal membranous transformation[2] (Figure 15.5). With more extensive glomerular involvement, hyaline eosinophilic deposits become more obvious and are distributed particularly along the inner aspects of the basement membrane and in the mesangium, so that the tufts gradually become less cellular and capillary lumina are obliterated (Figure 15.6). Special stains help to distinguish the amyloid deposits from those seen in advanced glomerulonephritis or diabetic nephropathy (Figure 15.7).

Tubular atrophy may be marked, particularly in advanced cases with peritubular and interstitial amyloid deposition. Intra-renal vessels, particularly interlobular arteries and arterioles, are generally involved in renal amyloidosis which is particularly marked in the medial and adventitial coats. In some primary forms, particularly that complicating myelomatosis, amyloid deposition may be confined to blood vessels.

Thrombosis of renal veins and their major tributaries may complicate any disease giving rise to the nephrotic syndrome and is a particular complication of renal amyloidosis.

Myelomatosis

Plasmacytic proliferative disorders include: (1) solitary myeloma of bone, (2) extramedullary plasmacytoma, (3) diffuse myelomatosis with widespread involvement of the bone marrow without tumour formation, (4) multiple myelomatosis with osteolytic lesions in bone, and (5) plasma cell leukaemia. These conditions are characterized by excessive immunoglobulin production. The immunoglobulins, which may belong to any of the major classes, are chemically and electrophoretically indistinguishable from those normally present. In an affected individual, however, a specific immunoglobulin and/or immunoglobulin fragment is produced throughout the course of their disease. This suggests that the proliferating plasma cells manufacturing the immunoglobulin are the progeny of a single precursor cell, a concept enshrined in the term 'monoclonal gammopathies'[3] which has been applied to these disorders.

Multiple myelomatosis is the commonest variant

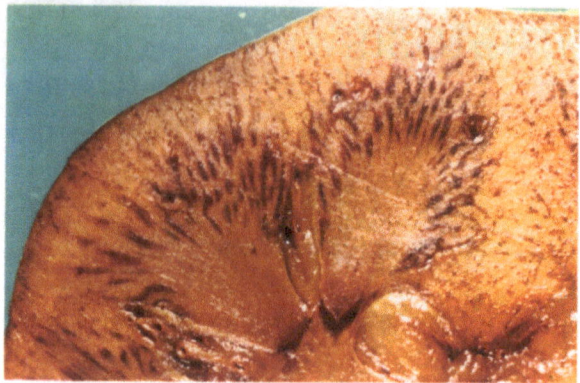

Figure 15.1   Renal amyloidosis. Macroscopic appearance of the cut surface of the kidney stained with iodine solution.

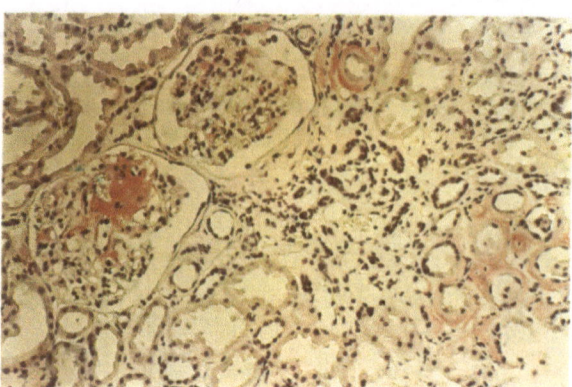

Figure 15.2   Renal amyloidosis. An area of renal cortex stained by Congo red to show deposition of amyloid in an arteriole, glomeruli and around several tubules.   × 240.

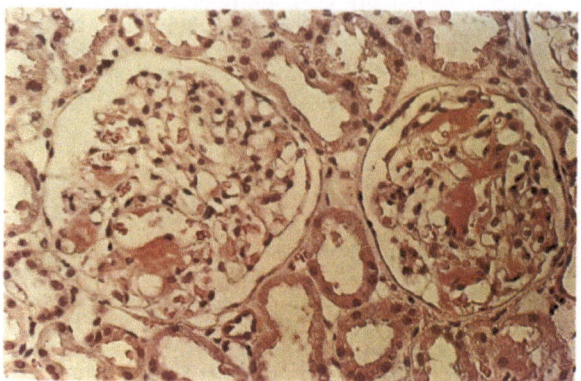

Figure 15.3   Renal amyloidosis. Two glomeruli showing amyloid deposits irregularly distributed. Congo red   × 360.

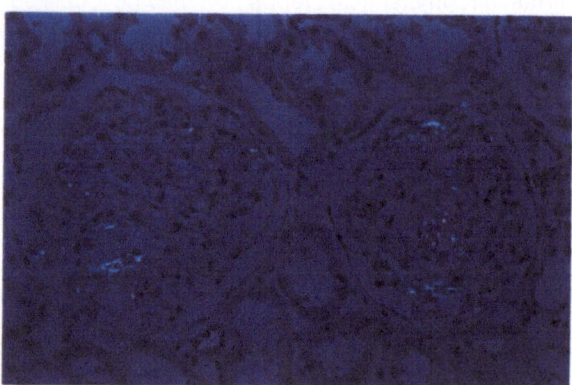

Figure 15.4   Renal amyloidosis. Identical field shown in Figure 15.2 but viewed by polarized light to show green birefringence of amyloid deposits. Congo red   × 360.

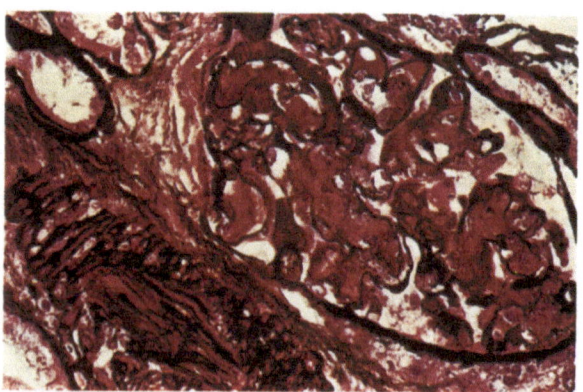

Figure 15.5   Renal amyloidosis. Deposition of amyloid on the epithelial aspects of some capillary loops with a sun-ray pattern of argyrophilia giving an appearance which resembles focal membranous transformation. H & E/ Methenamine silver   × 600.

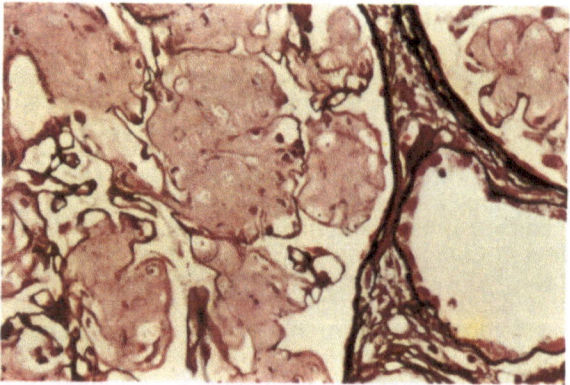

Figure 15.6   Renal amyloidosis. More advanced amyloidosis showing well-defined homogeneous eosinophilic deposits of amyloid largely within the confines of the glomerular capillary basement membrane. Unlike the nodules of diabetic glomerulosclerosis these large amyloid deposits lack argyrophilia. H & E/Methenamine silver   × 1020.

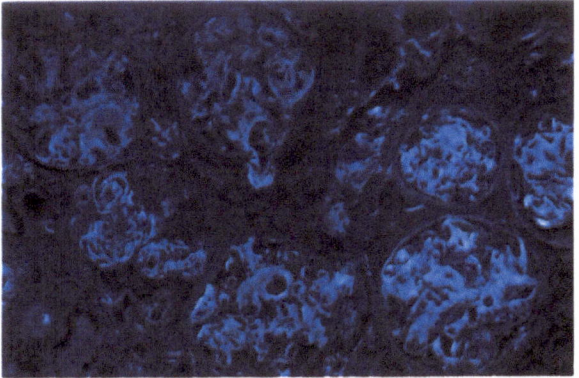

Figure 15.7 Renal amyloidosis. Extensive glomerular and arteriolar amyloid deposition demonstrated by UV fluorescence following thioflavine-T treatment. This case is one of those originally described by Richard Bright. The patient was a young woman of 25 years, who developed a nephrotic syndrome due to renal amyloidosis complicated extensive pulmonary tuberculosis. × 240.

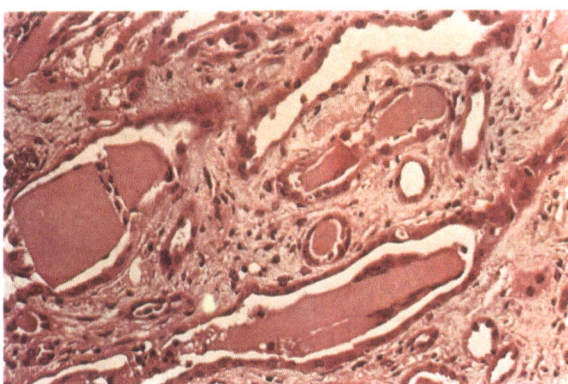

Figure 15.8 Myelomatosis. The renal tubules contain sharply defined, rather square-ended casts, one of which is associated with a syncytial collection of tubular epithelial cells. H & E × 600.

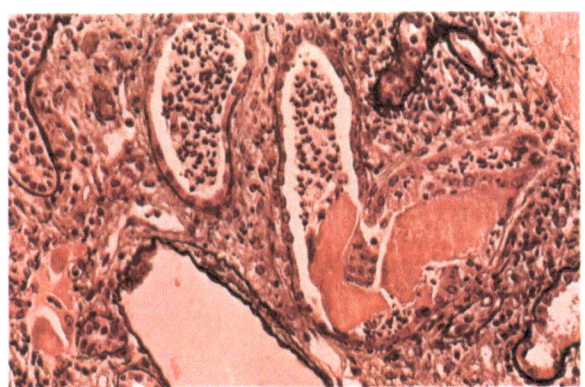

Figure 15.9 Myelomatosis. A tubular cast together with polymorphonuclear leukocytes filling the tubular lumen. The polymorphs probably reflect renal infection. H & E × 600.

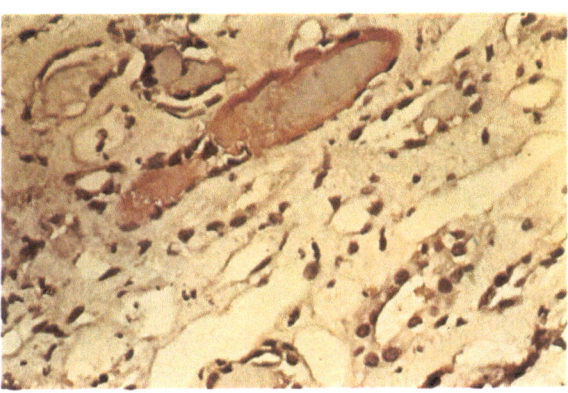

Figure 15:10 Myelomatosis. A tubular cast stained by Congo red to demonstrate amyloid deposition around its periphery. Congo red × 960.

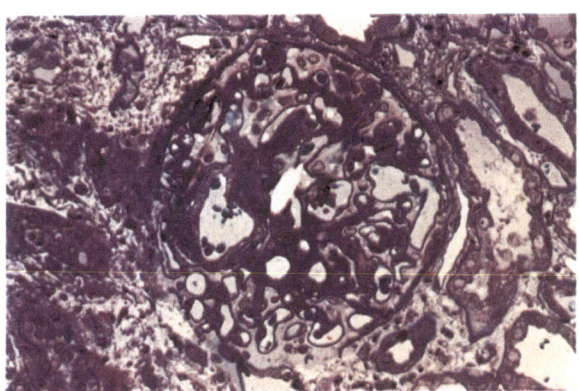

Figure 15.11 Myelomatosis. A glomerulus showing mesangial increase and prominence of the tuft loops reminiscent of early diabetic glomerulosclerosis. Plastic-embedded section; toluidine blue × 600.

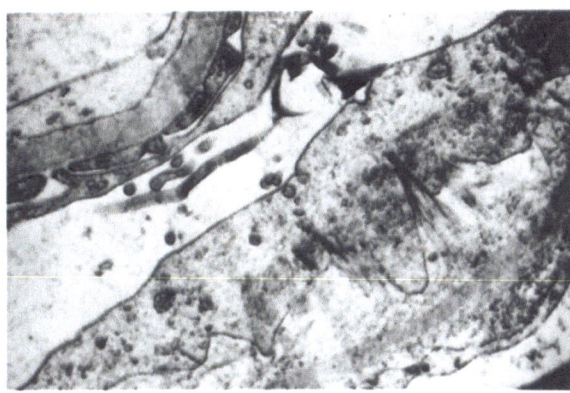

Figure 15.12 Renal amyloidosis. An electron micrograph showing spicular deposits of amyloid on the epithelial aspect of the basement membrane, covered by a thickened layer of epithelial cell cytoplasm. On light microscopy with silver impregnation, this pattern of amyloid deposition gives an appearance similar to membranous transformation. See Figure 15.5. × 3500.

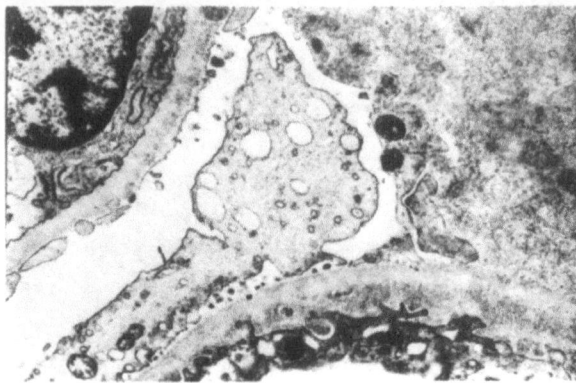

Figure 15.13 Renal amyloidosis. An electron micrograph showing a large nodular deposit limited on one side by epithelial cell cytoplasm. In the lower part of the picture amyloid deposition has occurred diffusely beneath the endothelial lining of a capillary loop and also within the basement membrane. × 5350.

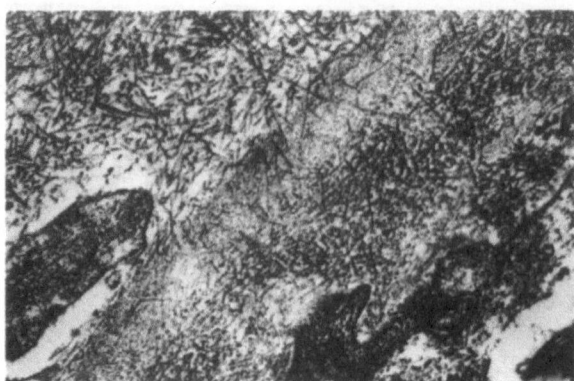

Figure 15.14 Renal amyloidosis. A high power electron micrograph of the same case illustrated in Figure 15.13, showing the fibrillary pattern of the amyloid protein with a matted mass of fibrils irregularly distributed. × 20 000.

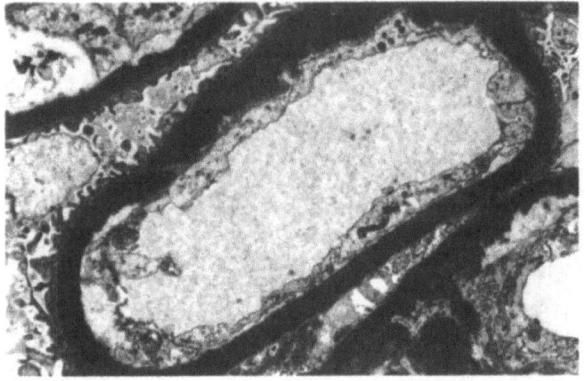

Figure 15.15 Myelomatosis. An electron micrograph showing diffuse thickening of the glomerular capillary basement membrane by an electron-dense material. Similar material is also present in the mesangium. × 4900.

and renal damage often occurs in this condition. About 50–60% of patients elaborate excessive light chain subunits of the immunoglobulin as well as the immunoglobulin itself. The light chains, because of their relatively small molecular weight, appear in the urine (Bence Jones protein). This is identified by the fact that it coagulates at temperatures between 45°C and 55°C and redissolves at higher temperatures.

One of the most characteristic features of the renal changes in multiple myelomatosis is the presence of casts in the tubules, particularly distal tubules and collecting ducts. These are brightly eosinophilic with a homogeneous hyaline or laminated appearance and occasionally a bluish tinge due to calcification (Figures 15.8 and 15.9). The casts are probably derived by precipitation of the abnormal proteins, and their presence correlates well with that of Bence Jones proteinuria[4]. Sometimes amyloid has been demonstrated in the tubular casts[5], particularly at their peripheries (Figure 15.10). Tubular dilatation, atrophy and loss, presumably due to obstruction by the casts, is frequently found and is probably the chief factor responsible for renal functional impairment. Around the casts themselves, the tubular epithelial cells frequently form syncytial giant cells. Occasionally

small needle-shaped crystals have been described in proximal tubular cells[6] and these too are presumably derived from abnormal proteins.

The glomeruli are usually normal, or show non-specific 'ischaemic' changes. Occasionally there is diffuse mesangial thickening and prominence of tuft capillary loops (Figure 15.15). This thickening does not appear to be amyloid, which is only rarely seen in the glomeruli in multiple myelomatosis, since it lacks the typical tinctoral and ultrastructural properties of amyloid. The thickening is probably related to the large protein load crossing the glomerular filter (Figure 15.11).

Because of the osteolytic lesions in multiple myelomatosis considerable amounts of calcium may be released causing hypercalcaemia and often calcium deposition in the kidneys, particularly in tubules and interstitial tissues. Pyelonephritis is also an occasional complication, perhaps related to the increased susceptibility to infection occurring in multiple myelomatosis. Systemic amyloidosis as a result of multiple myelomatosis has been referred to already. Its incidence is probably about 10–15% although renal involvement is much less common, and when it occurs is usually confined to blood vessels or occasionally to the tubular casts.

References

1. Leader (1979). Pathogenesis of amyloid disease. *Br. Med. J.,* **1**, 216.

2. Ansell, I. D. and Joekes, A. M. (1972). Spicular arrangement of amyloid in renal biopsy. *J. Clin. Pathol.,* **25**, 1056–1062.

3. Cohen, S. (1968). The nature of myeloma proteins. *Br. J. Haematol.,* **15**, 211–215.

4. Zinneman, H. H., Glenchur, H. and Gleason, D. F. (1960). The significance of urine electrophoresis in patients with multiple myeloma. *Arch. Intern. Med.,* **106**, 172–178.

5. Limas, C., Wright, J. R., Matsuzaki, M. and Calkins, E. (1973). Amyloidosis and multiple myeloma: a reevaluation using a control population. *Am. J. Med.,* **54**, 166–177.

6. Siki, H. (1949). A case of diffuse plasmacytosis with deposition of protein crystals in the kidneys. *J. Pathol. Bacteriol.,* **61**, 149–163.

The authors are grateful to Dr I. D. Ansell for providing Figure 15.12.

Diabetic Renal Disease and Urolithiasis

16

Renal abnormalities which may complicate diabetes mellitus include diabetic glomerulosclerosis, pyelonephritis, necrotizing papillitis and an increased incidence of arteriosclerosis.

Diabetic Glomerulosclerosis

This lesion is considered to be specific to diabetes; its incidence increases with the duration of diabetes and it is most prevalent in patients whose diabetes starts at an early age. There is some evidence that good control of the diabetes lessens the incidence of glomerulosclerosis. Clinically, proteinuria is usually present and a nephrotic syndrome develops in about 10% of cases. Two main types of glomerular change are described; the diffuse and the nodular (or Kimmelstiel–Wilson) lesions; often the two forms occur together. The diffuse lesion consists of widespread thickening of capillary walls and a moderate increase in mesangial matrix material (Figure 16.1). The capillary wall thickening, although diffuse, is seldom as uniform as in membranous glomerulonephritis. In the nodular lesions, rounded, homogeneous, eosinophilic accumulations of mesangial matrix are seen in the mesangial regions at the centres of glomerular tuft lobules (Figure 16.2). These nodules often vary in size and affect a varying proportion of glomeruli and of lobules within glomeruli. This contrasts with the lobular stage of mesangio-capillary glomerulonephritis in which mesangial nodularity is more uniformly distributed. Frequently the diffuse and nodular lesions of diabetic glomerulosclerosis occur together and it is very likely that they represent different aspects of a similar process.

Other glomerular changes seen in diabetes include the exudative (or fibrin cap) lesion and the capsular drop. The exudative lesion is a brightly eosinophilic, homogeneous deposit which forms within the concavity of tuft capillaries usually at the periphery of the tuft (Figures 16.3 and 16.4). This deposit stains red with Masson's trichrome and MSB, purple with phosphotungstic acid/haematoxylin and also in frozen sections with fat stains such as Sudan IV. It is not specific for diabetic glomerulosclerosis and is seen, for example, in severe nephrosclerosis, in various types of glomerulonephritis and in 'minimal change' disease following prolonged steroid therapy.

The capsular drop is a small rounded eosinophilic mass which is situated between the basement membrane and the epithelial cell lining of Bowman's capsule (Figure 16.5).

Arteriosclerosis and arteriolar sclerosis are almost always seen in diabetic nephrosclerosis and severe hyaline thickening of afferent and even efferent arterioles is particularly characteristic (Figure 16.3). A varying degree of tubular atrophy, depending on the extent of the glomerular and vascular lesions, is nearly always apparent even in small biopsy specimens. Chronic inflammatory cell infiltration, usually with a focal distribution, is generally present in the interstitium and should not necessarily be regarded as evidence of renal infection.

By electron microscopy the diffuse lesion shows widespread thickening of the basement membrane (up to ten times normal) and deposits of basement membrane-like material in the mesangium (Figure 16.6). The nocular lesion consists of large areas of similar basement membrane-like material within the mesangium and continuous with the adjacent glomerular basement membrane.

Results with immunofluorescence microscopy have been variable but sometimes linear deposits of immunoglobulins, complement components, fibrin, albumen, and other proteins such as insulin and caeruloplasmin have been described along the glomerular basement membrane. It is likely, in view of the inconsistency of these findings, that these deposits indicate non-specific adherence of plasma-derived components to the abnormally permeable basement membrane.

The pathogenesis of diabetic glomerulosclerosis has not been established. Lendrum et al.[1] regarded the hyaline deposits as accumulations of fibrin products altered by ageing which originally seeped from the capillaries as a result of the increased vascular permeability associated with diabetes. Other workers consider the basement membrane thickening and mesangial deposition of basement membrane-like material to reflect abnormal basement membrane synthesis related to the defects in carbohydrate metabolism in diabetes[2].

Pyelonephritis and Necrotizing Papillitis

It is usually accepted that there is an increased susceptibility to renal infections, both acute and chronic, in diabetes mellitus. Clinical surveys of the incidence of significant bacteriuria in ambulatory diabetic subjects, however, show no increase in urinary infections amongst young patients of either sex, and in older patients only amongst females[3-5]. The evidence for an increased incidence of chronic pyelonephritis in diabetics rests heavily on autopsy surveys[6,7] performed at a time when the finding of interstitial chronic inflammatory cell infiltration was accepted too uncritically as evidence of chronic infection, and it is probable that much of the change so interpreted was a reflection of vascular disease alone.

The incidence of acute pyelonephritis at autopsy

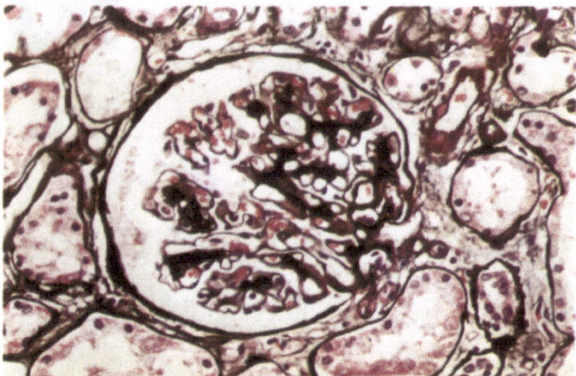

Figure 16.1 Diabetic glomerulosclerosis. The 'diffuse lesion' showing widespread thickening of glomerular capillary walls and an increase in mesangial matrix. H & E/Methenamine silver × 480.

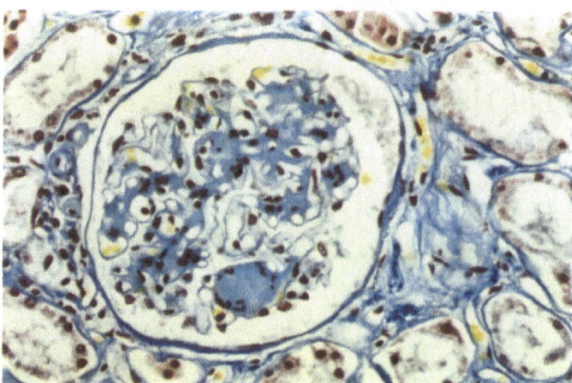

Figure 16.2 Diabetic glomerulosclerosis. Combined 'diffuse' and 'nodular' lesions. The nodule is rounded, acellular and homogeneous and occupies the centre of a lobule inferiorly. MSB × 480.

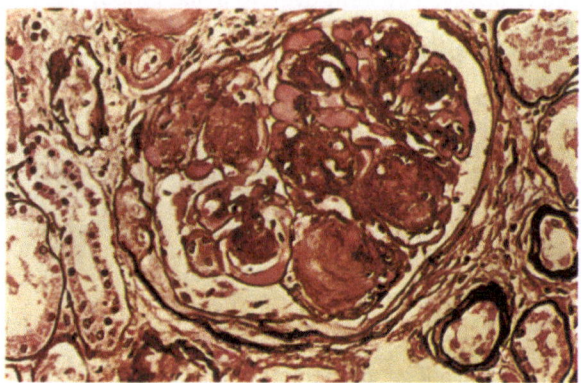

Figure 16.3 Diabetic glomerulosclerosis. A glomerulus showing advanced changes. Many of the tuft capillaries have homogeneous eosinophilic deposits within their concavities, characteristic of the 'exudative' or 'fibrin cap' lesion. At the top left, part of the afferent and the efferent artioles are seen, both showing hyaline arteriolosclerosis. H & E/Methenamine silver × 480.

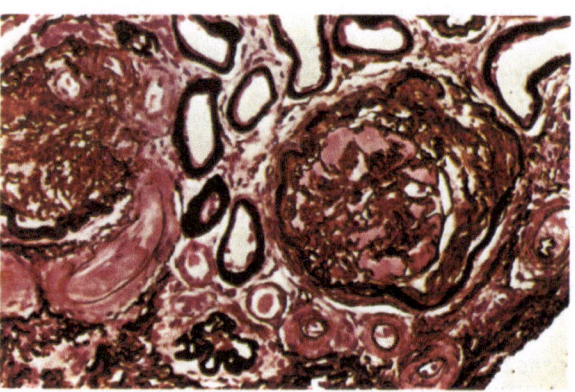

Figure 16.4 Diabetic glomerulosclerosis. Even in this glomerulus which is extensively sclerosed 'fibrin cap' lesions are readily seen. H & E/Methenamine silver × 480.

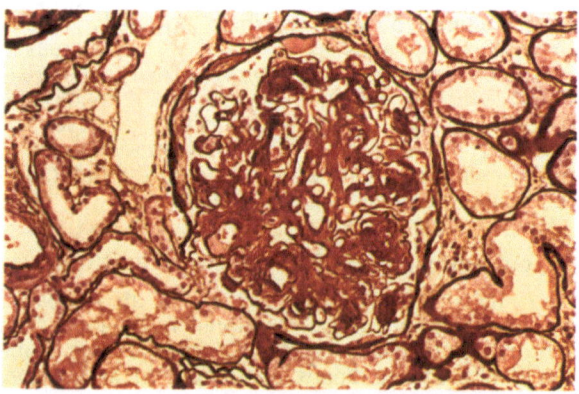

Figure 16.5 Diabetic glomerulosclerosis. A glomerulus showing advanced change with a 'capsular drop' lesion adherent to Bowman's capsule at 12 o'clock. H & E/Methenamine silver × 480.

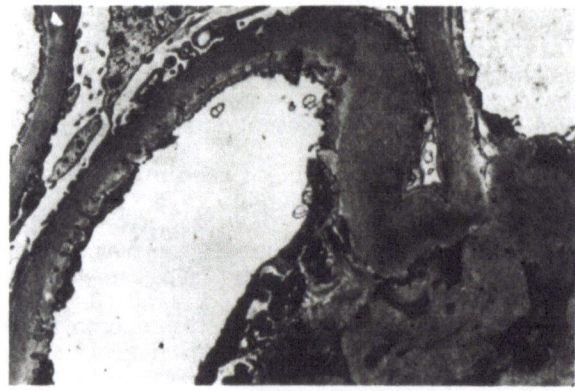

Figure 16.6 Diabetic glomerulosclerosis. An electron micrograph showing diffuse thickening of the basement membrane and deposits of similar material in the mesangium. × 5350.

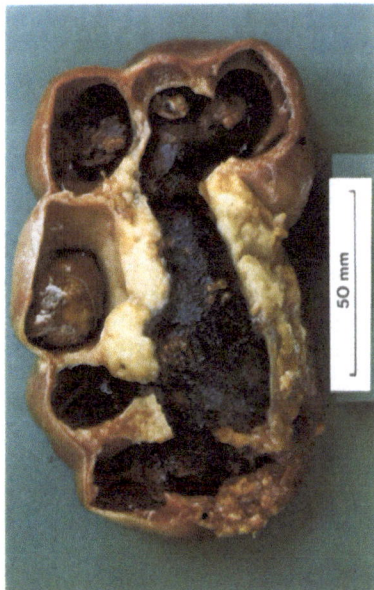

Figure 16.7 Urolithiasis. A 'staghorn' calculus filling the renal pelvis and calyceal system. There is generalized renal atrophy.

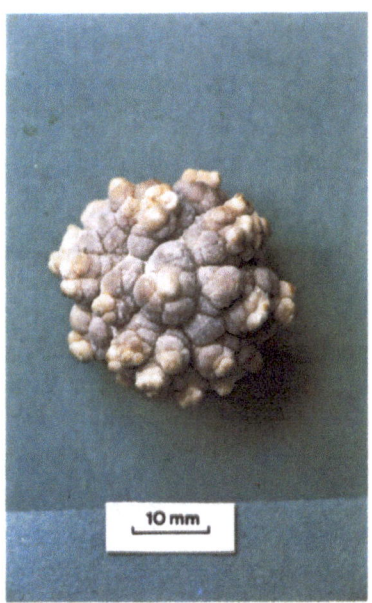

Figure 16.8 Urolithiasis. A mulberry stone composed of calcium oxalate. The surface is blackened by altered blood.

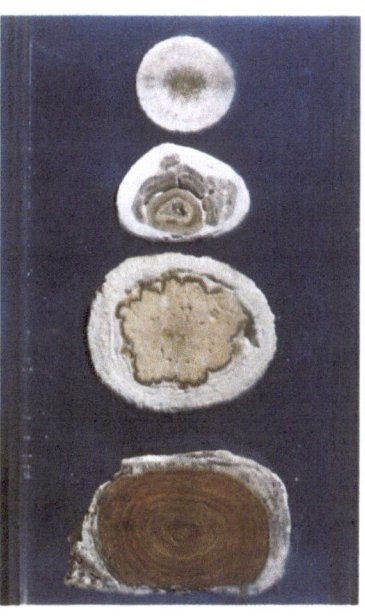

Figure 16.9 Urolithiasis. A collection of mixed calculi with centres of varying composition but all covered by calcium phosphate and triple phosphates.

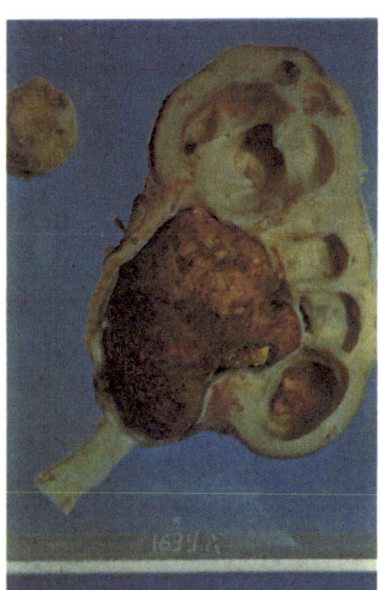

Figure 16.10 Urolithiasis. A kidney with a large calcium oxalate/phosphate stone filling the renal pelvis. The patient had hypercalcaemia and hypercalciuria due to a parathyroid adenoma which is shown top left.

is undoubtedly increased in diabetics, but in view of the information from population surveys of urinary infection in diabetics already referred to, this usually appears to be a late complication in terminally ill patients.

Acute papillary necrosis is a complication of acute pyelonephritis in diabetics and is more common in females and in those with co-existent diabetic glomerulosclerosis[8].

Urolithiasis

Calculi occur at any level in the urinary tract, the incidence in the various sites differing in different parts of the world. In Great Britain upper tract stones in the pelvi-calyceal system are the most common.

Stones are composed of crystalloids bound by a complex mucoprotein matrix. Phosphate stones composed of a mixture of calcium phosphate and triple phosphates are the most common variety. They are off-white or grey in colour, smooth and generally crumbly. Often such calculi fill the pelvi-calyceal system creating a 'cast' of it (the so-called 'staghorn' calculus; Figure 16.7). Calcium oxalate stones are also common. They are hard, with a spiny exterior (the 'mulberry' stone) and are discoloured dark brown or black externally due to blood staining (Figure 16.8). Stones composed of uric acid alone or a mixture of uric acid and phosphate are less common (Figure 16.9). They are moderately hard and yellow-brown in colour. Cystine and xanthine stones are rare; cystine stones, which are usually multiple, are small, smooth, round, and yellow.

The mechanisms of stone formation are poorly understood. Urine is a complex mixture of many substances including crystalloids present in concentrations which in normal aqueous solution would be supersaturated. It is thought that the various colloidal components of urine help to maintain the crystalloids in solution, and disturbances in the balance between them may precipitate stone formation. Changes in urine pH may be important in this respect. Both uric acid and cystine are much less soluble at low pH values and stones composed of these substances tend to form in acid urine. Conversely phosphate stones form in alkaline urine. They are frequently associated with urinary infections by urea-splitting organisms such as *Proteus* in which urinary pH is kept high by the release of ammonia. Dehydration is another important factor as shown by the often almost epidemic incidence of renal stones in troops recently arrived in the tropics.

Excessive urinary excretion of the various constituent crystalloids is also associated with an increased incidence of stone formation. Hypercalcuria may occur idiopathically or as a complication of hyperparathyroidism (Figure 16.10), sarcoidosis, Cushing's syndrome, multiple myelomatosis, prolonged immobilization, primary renal tubular acidosis or the milk–alkali syndrome. Primary hyperoxaluria, as well as causing calcium oxalate deposits throughout the body, is associated with calcium oxalate stone formation. However, most patients with oxalate stones do not have primary hyperoxaluria and no increased urinary oxalate excretion can be demonstrated. Gout causes a high urinary uric acid excretion and is associated with uric acid stone formation particularly when the urine is acid. In practice, only about 25% of patients with uric acid stones have gout. Cystine and xanthine stones occur exclusively in the rare metabolic disorders cystinuria and xanthinuria.

Local factors are also thought to be important in stone formation. A nucleus of organic or crystalloid material can often be identified at the centres of renal calculi and it is probable that small pieces of blood clot, fibrin, cellular debris or collections of bacteria, etc. can act as a nidus around which crystals can form and initiate stone formation. Tiny foci of calcification (Randall's plaques) can occasionally be identified near collecting ducts at the tips of the renal pyramids, and these have also been suggested as possible starting points for stone formation. It should be stressed, however, that Randall's plaques are common even in patients who do not form stones, and are by no means universal in patients with stones.

References

1. Lendrum, A. C., Fraser, D. S., Slidders, W. and Henderson, R. (1962). Studies on the character and staining of fibrin. *J. Chem. Pathol.*, **15**, 401–413.

2. Beisswenger, P. J. and Spiro, R. G. (1970). Human glomerular basement membrane: chemical alteration in diabetes mellitus. *Science*, **168**, 596–598.

3. Kass, E. H. (1960). Bacteriuria and the pathogenesis of pyelonephritis. *Lab. Invest.*, **9**, 110–116.

4. Vejlsgaard, R. (1966). Studies on urinary infection in diabetics: II. Significant bacteriuria in relation to long-term diabetic manifestation. *Acta Med. Scand.*, **179**, 183–188.

5. Pometta, D., Rees, S. B., Younger, D. and Kass, E. H. (1967). Asymptomatic bacteriuria in diabetes mellitus. *N. Engl. J. Med.*, **276**, 1118–1121.

6. Aarseth, S. (1953). Cardiovascular renal disease in diabetes mellitus. *Acta Med. Scand.*, **281** (Suppl.).

7. Young, K. R. and Clancy, C. F. (1955). Urinary tract infections complicating diabetes mellitus. *Med. Clin. N. Am.*, **39**, 1665–1670.

8. Edmondson, H. A., Martin, H. E. and Evans, N. (1947). Necrosis of renal papillae and acute pyelonephritis in diabetes mellitus. *Arch. Intern. Med.*, **79**, 148–179.

Renal transplantation is now an accepted treatment for end-stage renal disease. Most donor kidneys are cadaver allografts, but grafts from close living relatives are also used and the best results are obtained with isografts from identical twins. Although many patients make good progress following transplantation, a number of factors may affect graft function particularly during the first three months. These are more frequently a problem with cadaver kidneys than with grafts from living donors, and include poor preservation of the donor kidney, allograft rejection, vascular and ureteric complications due to causes other than rejection, infection of the graft, and rarely recurrence of the recipient's original disease.

Prior to transplantation, tests are made of ABO compatibility and for the presence in the recipient of pre-existing antibodies against donor HLAs (human lymphocyte antigens) by crossmatching recipient serum with donor lymphocytes. Incompatibilities of either nature can result in hyperacute graft rejection and are therefore absolute contraindications for transplantation. Two loci (the A and B) of the HLA system can be tested routinely in most centres, and D locus compatibility can be tested by mixed lymphocyte culture (MLC). Donors are selected on the basis of the best available match to minimize as far as possible histo-incompatibility, although obviously this cannot be entirely eliminated. Immunosuppressive therapy is given routinely following transplantation and rejection episodes are treated by increased dosages of these drugs.

Renal biopsy in transplanted patients is indicated under the following circumstances:

(1) Anuria following transplantation for longer than two weeks.

(2) Following clinical evidence of rejection where no response to increased immunosuppressive treatment occurs.

(3) Slowly deteriorating renal function.

(4) Increased proteinuria and/or haematuria.

Hyperacute Rejection

This type of rejection occurs in the majority of patients with major ABO incompatibility and in about 80% of patients with preformed cytotoxic antibodies to donor lymphocytes. Macroscopic changes in the kidney (softening and bluish mottling of the surface) are usually evident at operation 10 to 20 minutes after the graft has been inserted. Cortical necrosis is evident within a day or two (Figure 17.1). Microscopically fibrin and platelet thrombi block many glomerular and peritubular capillaries and neutrophil polymorphonuclear leukocytes line the capillary walls (Figures 17.2 and 17.3). By electron microscopy platelet aggregates fill many capillary lumina and by immunofluorescence microscopy linear localization of IgG and C3 is seen on capillary walls.

Acute Rejection

Most patients with renal allografts undergo one or more clinical episodes of acute rejection despite continuous immunosuppressive therapy. These episodes are commonest during the first few weeks after transplantation and are rare after a year. Renal biopsy is usually only performed if a satisfactory response is not obtained to increased dosage of immunosuppressive agents. Two principal varieties of change may be seen:

Predominantly Cellular Rejection

This is characterized by a diffuse, but usually focally accentuated cellular infiltration of an oedematous interstitium (Figure 17.4). This contains mononuclear cells — lymphocytes, pyroninophilic immunoblasts, plasma cells and histiocytes. Mitotic figures amongst the lymphoid cells are not infrequent. The intertubular capillaries are congested and the swollen endothelial lining cells are often lifted from the basement membrane by lymphoid cells. Focal breaks in the endothelial basement membrane can frequently be observed even by light microscopy. The infiltrate is often dense beneath the tubular epithelium and focal necrosis and regeneration of tubular cells can be seen. Glomeruli and blood vessels are usually normal and immunofluorescence microscopy shows no glomerular deposition of immunoglobulin or complement.

Predominantly Vascular Rejection

Cellular infiltration is generally less marked and may even be absent. The lesion is characterized by foci of fibrinoid necrosis or intimal fibrin deposition in the walls of arterioles and small arteries (Figure 17.5) and sometimes fibrinoid necrosis of glomerular tufts. Platelet aggregates, often showing degranulation by electron microscopy, are prevalent within capillaries and small venules and may be associated with fibrin thrombi and neutrophil polymorphs adherent to the vessel walls. Interstitial haemorrhage and oedema and focal tubular necrosis may also be features. Immunofluorescence microscopy reveals immunoglobulins (IgG and IgM), complement components and fibrin in arteriolar walls, in peritubular capillaries and in a linear pattern

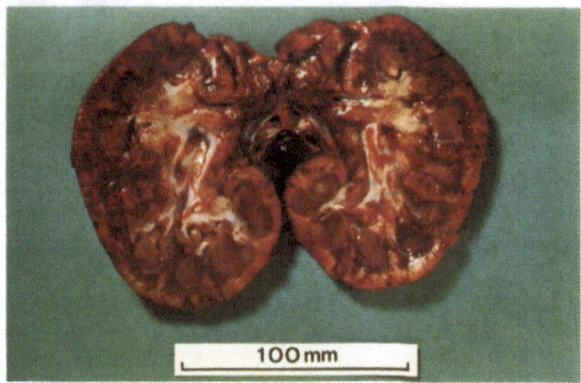

Figure 17.1   Hyperacute rejection. Extensive bilateral cortical necrosis in a transplant kidney removed after 2 days, following hyperacute rejection.

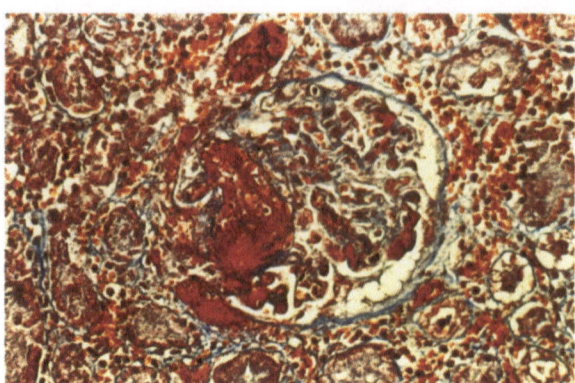

Figure 17.2   Hyperacute rejection. Segmental thrombosis, necrosis and fibrin deposition within a glomerular tuft. There is extensive interstitial haemorrhage. MSB   × 480.

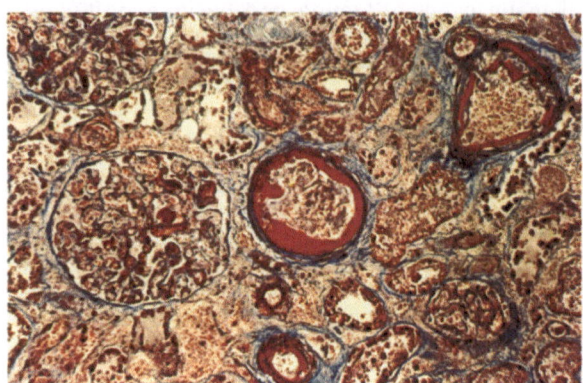

Figure 17.3   Hyperacute rejection. An area of cortical necrosis with fibrin/platelet thrombi occluding interlobular arteries and afferent arterioles. MSB   × 240.

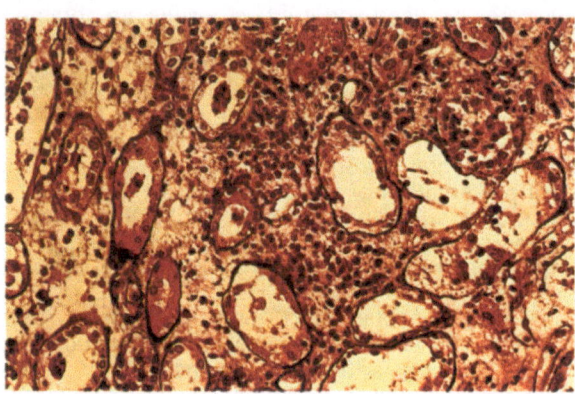

Figure 17.4   Acute rejection. Diffuse interstitial mononuclear cell infiltration with widespread tubular separation and oedema. There are variable degrees of tubular epithelial necrosis. H & E/Methenamine silver   × 240.

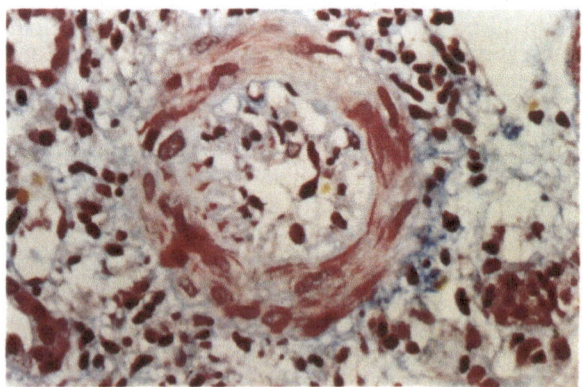

Figure 17.5   Acute rejection. An interlobular artery showing marked swelling and vacuolation of the endothelial cells, associated with fibrin deposition. MSB   × 600.

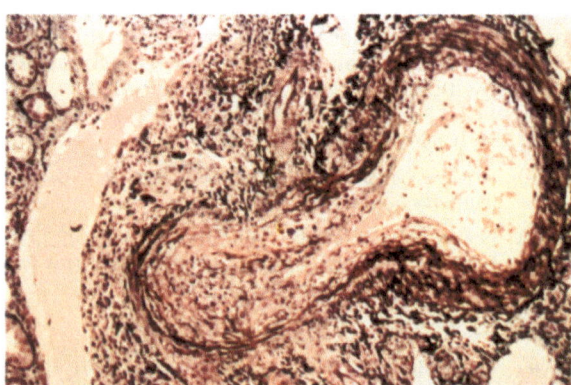

Figure 17.6 Acute on chronic rejection. Section showing the origin of an interlobular artery. As well as myo-intimal proliferation there is infiltration of the subintima by mononuclear cells, mainly lymphocytes. × 240.

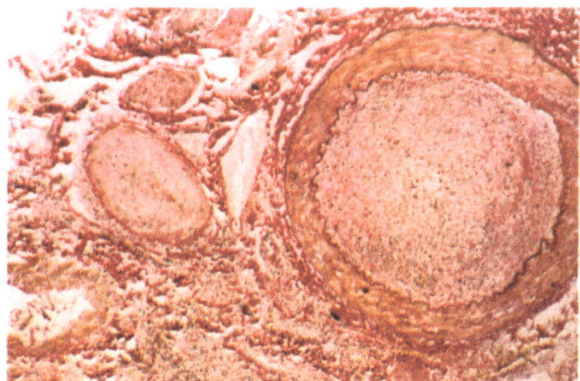

Figure 17.7 Chronic rejection. An arcuate and an interlobular artery showing pronounced proliferation of myo-intimal cells inside the internal elastic lamina. The vessels are almost completely occluded. Elastic Van Gieson × 240.

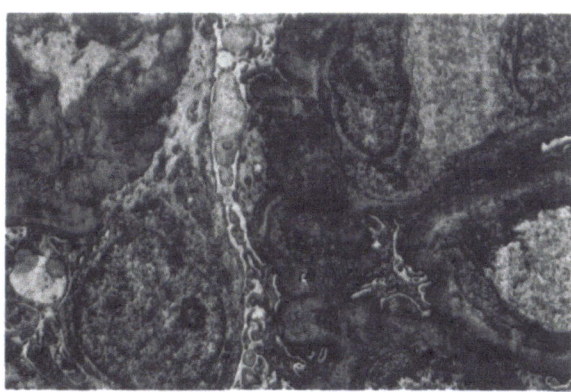

Figure 17.8 Chronic rejection. An electron micrograph showing thickening and wrinkling of the glomerular capillary basement membranes with some mesangial increase, and early mesangial interposition. The subendothelial zones are widened and relatively electron-lucent. × 3400.

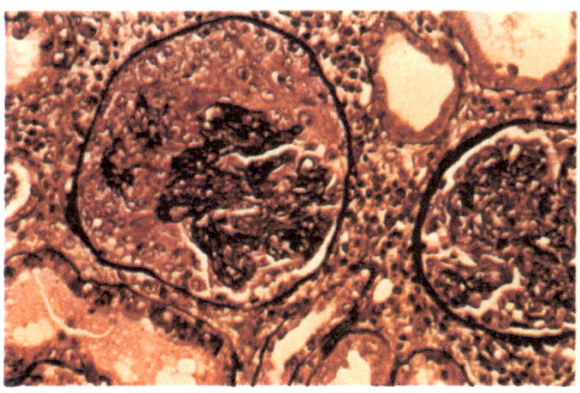

Figure 17.9 Recurrent glomerulonephritis in a transplant. An adult male patient with 'double contour' mesangiocapillary glomerulonephritis whose disease recurred in the transplant. One month after insertion of the graft, he developed a severe nephrotic syndrome and the transplanted kidney was removed after two months. The section of the renal transplant shows a large cellular crescent in one glomerulus and some interstitial mononuclear cell infiltration – probably indicating some cellular rejection. H & E/Methenamine silver × 480.

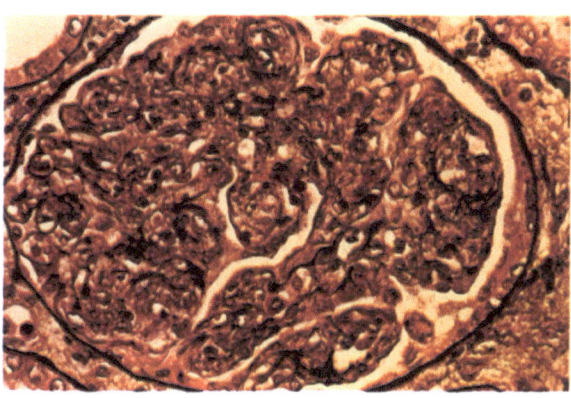

Figure 17.10 Recurrent glomerulonephritis in a transplant. A glomerulus from the renal transplant illustrated in Figure 17.9. This shows the typical changes of mesangiocapillary glomerulonephritis. H & E/Methenamine silver × 960.

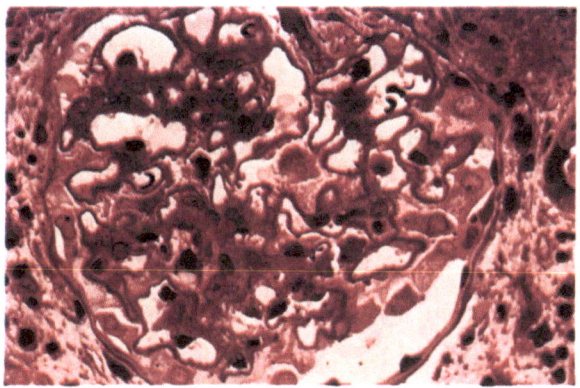

Figure 17.11 Recurrent glomerulonephritis in a transplant. A male child with 'dense deposit' mesangiocapillary glomerulonephritis who received a renal transplant which was biopsied 7 months after insertion. This plastic-embedded section of a glomerulus shows dense staining of the basement membranes of the glomerular tuft and Bowman's capsule. The changes are not typical of fully developed dense deposit disease. Toluidine blue × 960.

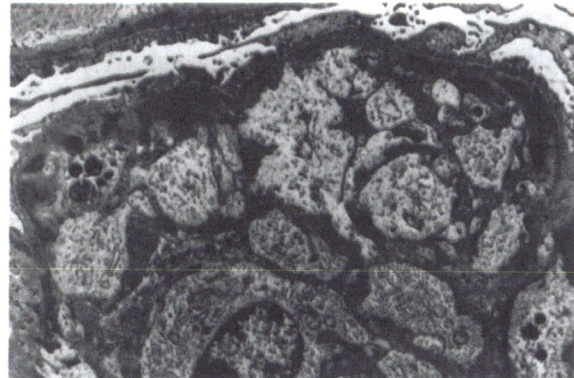

Figure 17.12 Recurrent glomerulonephritis in a transplant. An electron micrograph of a glomerulus from the same case illustrated in Figure 17.11. There is marked proliferation of mesangial cells and 'dense deposits' are present within the glomerular basement membrane. The lesion is not fully developed at this stage and this probably accounts for the light microscopy appearances. Recurrence of 'dense deposit' mesangiocapillary glomerulonephritis in renal transplants is almost invariable. × 6800.

along the glomerular basement membranes.

It is usually considered that the cellular form of acute rejection is mediated by cellular mechanisms whilst the vascular form is predominantly humoral. Herbertson et al.[1] have drawn attention to the prognostic significance of the various changes in acute allograft rejection and have shown that early graft failure correlates well with the presence of medial necrosis of arteries, acute glomerular lesions and interstitial haemorrhage. Less than 10% of grafts showing on biopsy one or more of these lesions, and none with all three, were capable of supporting life at 1 year. These authors also noted a significant association of subsequent poor graft function with the presence of mononuclear cell infiltration of the intima of arteries (Figure 17.6). No clear relationship was shown between interstitial cellular infiltration and subsequent graft survival. Tubular necrosis was also difficult to assess, particularly in very early biopsies when the change may merely represent ischaemic damage prior to graft insertion. It is probable that a better assessment of this change can be made by establishing its cause, although when extensive it is likely to indicate poor future performance.

Chronic Rejection

The principal change is a patchy progressive narrowing of arteries, usually most marked in those of arcuate and interlobular size (Figure 17.7). The narrowing is largely intimal, and is due to proliferation of myo-intimal and smooth muscle cells, the endothelial lining remaining intact. Breaks in the internal elastic lamina may be seen. Myo-intimal cells are often vacuolated and may contain conspicuous lipid deposits. Serial biopsies suggest that the thickening is due to gradual formation of platelet and fibrin aggregates in the vessel wall and then subsequent organization; by immunofluorescence microscopy deposits of IgM, complement and fibrin may be seen in the thickened intima. The arterial narrowing is accompanied by ischaemic atrophy of glomeruli and tubules, and interstitial fibrosis which is most marked in the peripheral cortex and may be accompanied by segmental areas of infarction.

The glomeruli, particularly in long-surviving allografts, show a variety of changes. In addition to purely ischaemic changes, there may be a diffuse or segmental thickening of some glomerular basement membranes and an increase in mesangial matrix sometimes accompanied by mesangial cell proliferation (Figure 17.8). Focal areas of tuft sclerosis, capsular adhesions and small reactive capsular crescents may also be features. By immunofluorescence microscopy, usually granular deposits of IgM, sometimes IgG and complement components may be seen along glomerular capillary loops and in the mesangium. Ultrastructurally amorphous deposits in the sub-endothelium and in the mesangium may be apparent. Similar deposits may also occur in arteriolar walls and occasionally in peritubular capillaries.

The changes of chronic rejection may occur surprisingly quickly and significant arterial thickening is occasionally seen within a few weeks of transplantation, when it probably represents a progression of the changes seen in acute vascular rejection. More commonly they are a later complication and are generally reflected clinically by a gradual deterioration in graft function.

Recurrence of Recipient's Original Disease in the Transplant

This is a rare phenomenon (see Table 17.1), although changes of recurrent chronic glomerulonephritis may be difficult to distinguish from those of chronic rejection (Figures 17.9, 17.10, 17.11 and 17.12).

Transmission of Disease from Graft to Host

Malignant disease has occasionally been transmitted via a renal allograft and may metastasize widely, possibly as a result of immunosuppressive therapy. For this reason patients with malignant disease should never be used as graft donors.

Various infections, including viral hepatitis, histoplasmosis and cryptococcosis have also been transmitted by allografts.

References

1. Herbertson, B. M., Evans, D. B., Calne, R. Y. and Banerjee, A. K. (1977). Percutaneous needle biopsies of renal allografts: the relationship between morphological changes present in biopsies and subsequent allograft function. Histopathology, **1**, 161–178.

Table 17.1   Recurrent host disease in transplanted kidney

1. *Glomerulonephritis*	
Diffuse endocapillary/mesangial proliferative glomerulonephritis	Very rare
Diffuse mesangiocapillary glomerulonephritis	
Double contour variety	Common
Dense deposit variety	Almost invariable
Diffuse membranous glomerulonephritis	Rare
Diffuse extracapillary glomerulonephritis	Frequent
Focal segmental proliferative glomerulonephritis	May occur in some types*
Focal segmental glomerulosclerosis	Moderately frequent
2. *Others*	
Metabolic diseases, particular oxalosis, and much less frequently cysteinosis, may be transmitted	

*Moderately frequent in IgA disease, occasional in some systemic disorders

Alport's Syndrome and Congenital Nephrotic Syndrome

Alport's Syndrome

Alport's syndrome was first described in 1927 and may be defined as an inherited, structural abnormality of glomerular capillary basement membranes together with one or more associated features. The structural abnormality of the glomerular basement membrane requires electron microscopy for accurate identification[1,2], although light microscopy may enable one to identify a range of non-specific abnormalities. More recently, it has been noted that anti-basement membrane antibody from patients with Goodpasture's syndrome will not bind to the glomeruli of patients with Alport's syndrome[3].

The best-known associated features of Alport's syndrome are deafness and progression to end-stage renal failure although neither may be present when the patient is first seen. Other less commonly associated features are ocular abnormalities such as anterior lenticonus, giant platelets, bony abnormalities, polyneuropathy and hyperprolinaemia. The initial presentation is usually with persistent microscopic haematuria often accompanied by some proteinuria; gross haematuria may follow an upper respiratory tract infection. Although detailed family studies have shown that the structural abnormality occurs more frequently in females they usually remain asymptomatic and rarely progress to chronic renal failure. A symptomatic patient is therefore likely to be a male child of around 7–10 years with normal renal function. If a renal biopsy is carried out at this stage, the findings are often misleadingly unimpressive. There may be some proliferation of mesangial cells, often varying in degree from one glomerulus to the next with a corresponding increase in mesangial matrix (Figures 18.1 and 18.2). We have been unimpressed by the suggestion that 'fetal'-type glomeruli with prominent epithelial cells are typical of Alport's syndrome despite the claims of some papers on this subject. Interstitial foam cells occur in about one-third of cases and are particularly suggestive of Alport's syndrome in the absence of a full nephrotic syndrome (Figure 18.3). No evidence of immune deposits can be found by immunochemical techniques, although patchy non-specific staining for IgM and C3 may occur. It is important to carry out electron microscopy on the glomeruli of all children with haematuria, mesangial proliferation and negative immunochemical investigations to confirm or exclude Alport's syndrome. Obviously the knowledge of a close relative with renal disease would make one suspicious, but one may be dealing with the first case to be identified in an affected family.

The structural abnormality seen by electron microscopy in its fully developed form is described as splitting and lamellation of the lamina densa of the glomerular capillary basement membranes (Figure 18.11). The outer layer of the lamina densa tends to form a series of irregular peaks (Figure 18.12), while the inner layer remains relatively smooth. Between the laminae, foci of dots and circles of varying sizes can be seen (Figure 18.13). This basement membrane abnormality needs to be generalized before a confident diagnosis of Alport's syndrome can be made. In children who have had renal biopsies performed at a very early age (under five years) the basement membranes appear very attenuated rather than lamellated. Since this is identical with the morphological features of the benign recurrent familial haematuria syndrome a definite diagnosis of Alport's syndrome may not be possible.

As the disease progresses the proteinuria increases and the patient may become overtly nephrotic. On light microscopy, foci of tubular atrophy, interstitial fibrosis and glomerular sclerosis may be identified; the latter being segmental, global or both (Figures 18.4, 18.5 and 18.6). Occasionally the proliferative change may be the more prominent and we have seen both segmental proliferative lesions and epithelial crescents in Alport's syndrome (Figures 18.7, 18.8 and 18.9).

The genetic inheritance of the disease is very complex which presumably means that more than one pair of gene loci are involved, and is probably best summarized as being a basic autosomal dominant pattern modified by incomplete penetrance in the female members of an affected family[4]. So far no satisfactory evidence has been documented of the transmission of the basement membrane abnormality to the graft of a renal transplant recipient.

Congenital Nephrotic Syndrome

The term congenital nephrotic syndrome is usually taken to refer to those cases in which children present with a severe nephrotic syndrome at or soon after birth[5]. Associated features include an enlarged placenta, high α-fetoprotein in the maternal amniotic fluid, and sometimes pyloric stenosis and congenital heart disease. The proteinuria may be highly selective at first and there may also be some haematuria. Histologically, little abnormality may be seen at first apart from foot process fusion by electron microscopy (Figure 18.14). There is a tendency for progressive sclerosis of glomeruli affecting the mesangial matrix together with some proliferation of mesangial cells in the Finnish type. Microcysts are described in the deep cortex and these probably represent dilated proximal convoluted tubules (Figure 18.10). The non-Finnish cases develop focal segmental sclerosing lesions within the glomeruli. Both varieties are resistant to treatment with

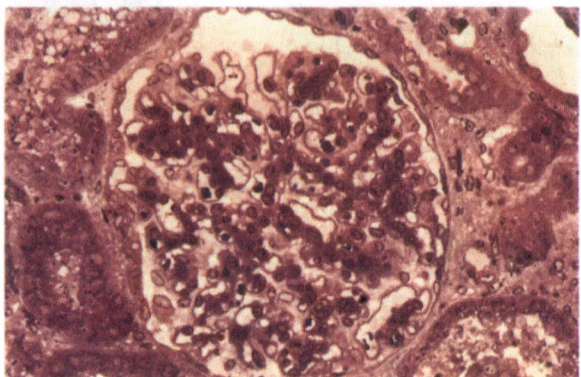

Figure 18.1   Alport's syndrome. An early glomerular lesion from a male child showing diffuse mesangial proliferation. Plastic-embedded section stained with toluidine blue   × 600.

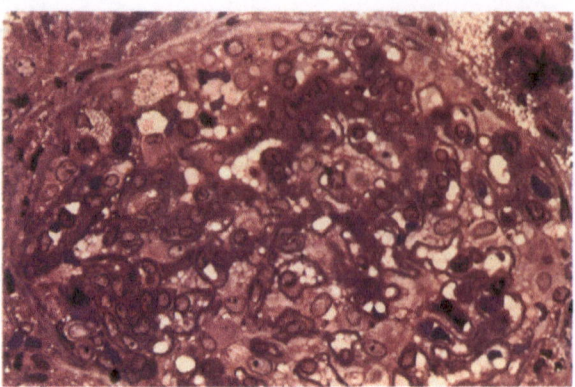

Figure 18.2   Alport's syndrome. Part of a glomerulus showing mainly mesangial proliferation. In the upper part, two epithelial foam cells with vacuolated cytoplasm are seen. Toluidine blue (plastic-embedded) × 1020.

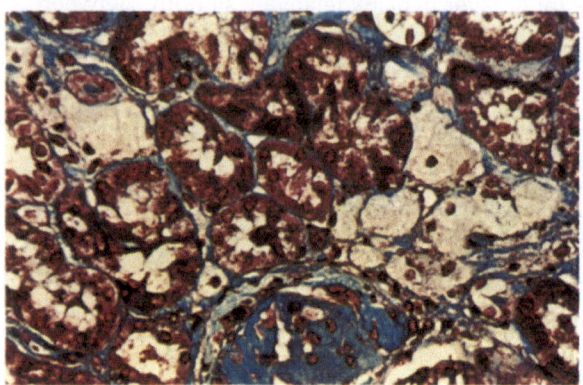

Figure 18.3   Alport's syndrome. Foam cells are present in the interstitium. In the absence of a nephrotic syndrome this feature is very suggestive of the diagnosis. Masson Trichrome stain   × 600.

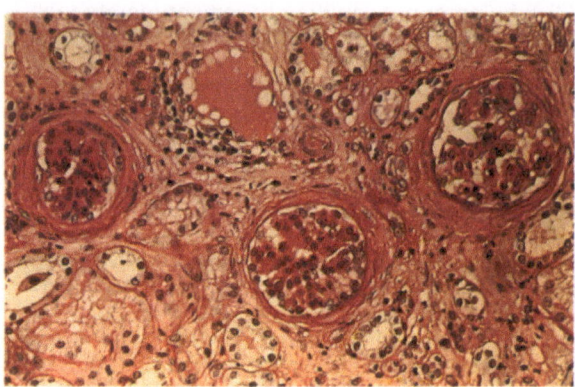

Figure 18.4   Alport's syndrome. A low power photomicrograph showing a variable degree of mesangial sclerosis, and interstitial fibrosis. PAS × 240.

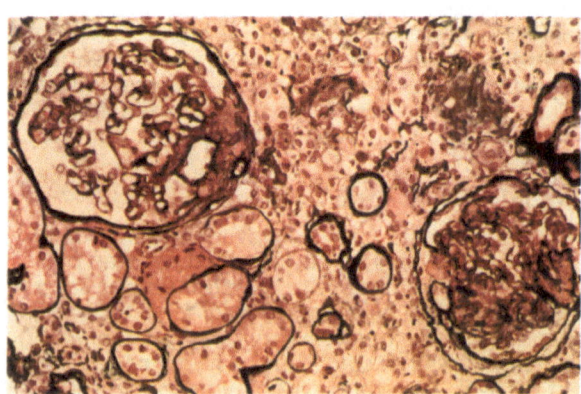

Figure 18.5   Alport's syndrome. The glomeruli show both segmental and global sclerosis and include some hyaline masses. H & E/Methenamine silver   × 360.

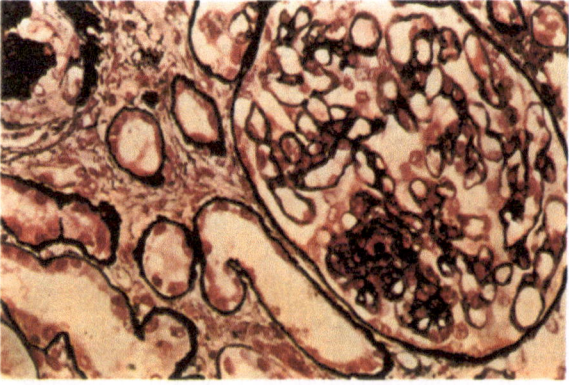

Figure 18.6   Alport's syndrome. A glomerulus showing segmental hyalinization. Elsewhere in the tuft the basement membrane is focally thickened and irregular. This feature is by no means specific, but may be a useful pointer. H & E/Methenamine silver   × 600.

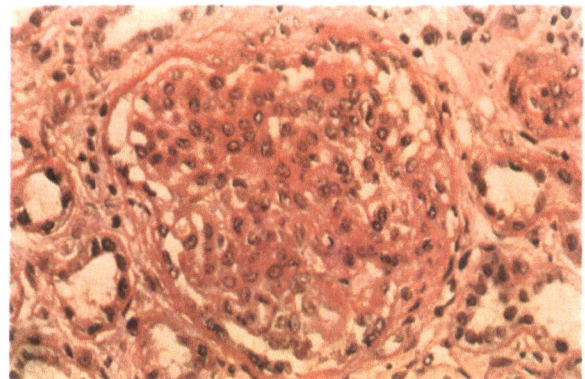

Figure 18.7 Alport's syndrome. A glomerulus showing proliferative change with some diffuse sclerosis and capsular adhesions. PAS × 600.

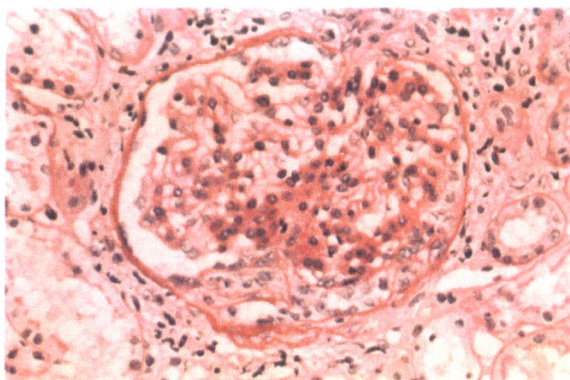

Figure 18.8 Alport's syndrome. Segmental proliferative change with some sclerosis. There is a capsular adhesion with some reactive epithelial cell proliferation. × 480.

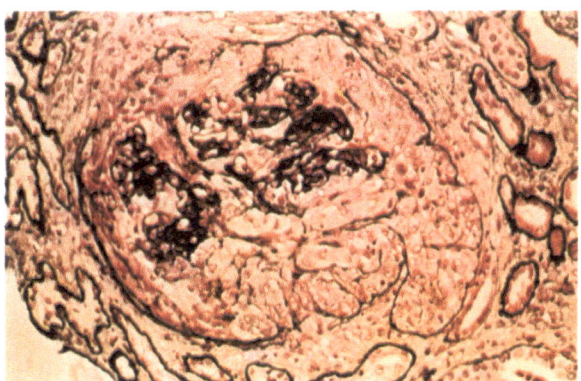

Figure 18.9 Alport's syndrome. A glomerulus showing florid capsular crescent formation. This is an occasional feature of the disease, but only a minority of glomeruli are usually affected. H & E/Methenamine silver × 600.

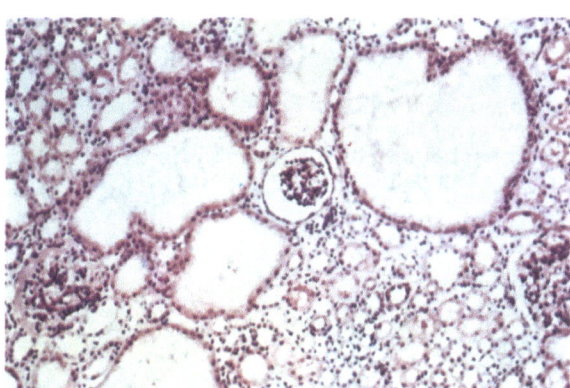

Figure 18.10 Congenital nephrotic syndrome. An area of deep cortex with microcystic change. H & E × 160.

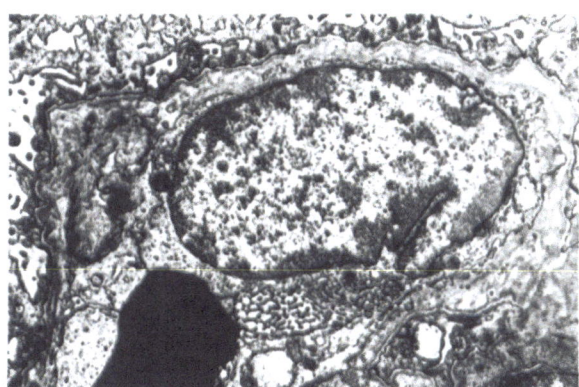

Figure 18.11 Alport's syndrome. Confirmation of the diagnosis which may be suspected on the clinical and light microscopic findings, requires electron microscopy. This electron micrograph shows some typical changes, namely marked splitting and lamellation of the lamina densa of the glomerular basement. × 6550.

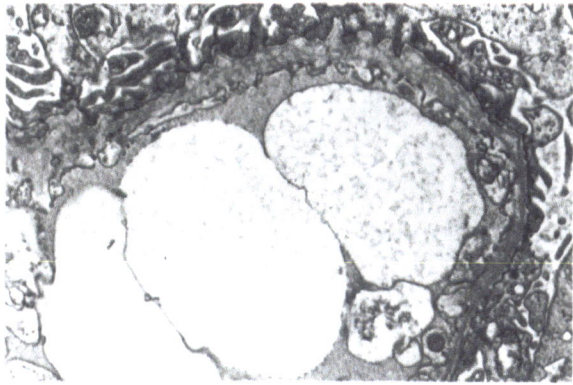

Figure 18.12 Alport's syndrome. An electron micrograph showing marked irregularity of the external contour of the basement membrane which could be misinterpreted as membranous transformation although there are no electron dense sub-epithelial deposits. × 6550.

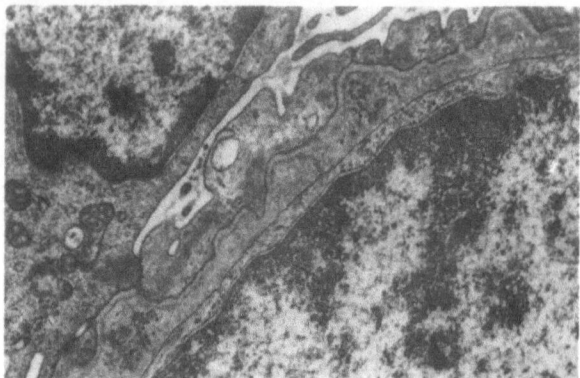

Figure 18.13 Alport's syndrome. A high power electron micrograph of the basement membrane showing the irregular external contour and groups of variable sized granules within the substance of the lamina densa. × 16 400.

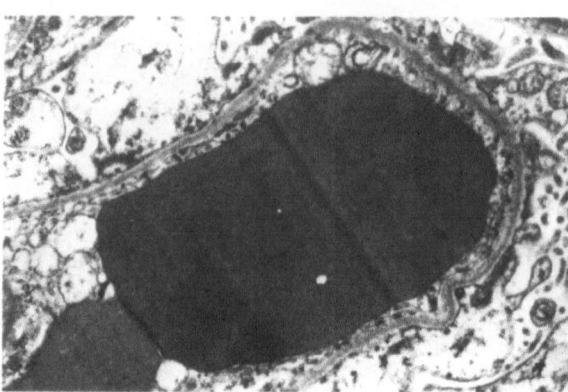

Figure 18.14 Congenital nephrotic syndrome. Part of a glomerulus from a newborn infant with this condition showing diffuse fusion of epithelial foot processes. × 7200.

steroids or cyclophosphamide and in the Finnish type many of the patients succumb to intercurrent infections before the disease has progressed to chronic renal failure.

References

1. Hill, G. S., Jenis, E. H. and Goodloe, S. (1974). The non-specificity of the ultrastructural alterations in hereditary nephritis: with additional observations on benign familial haematuria. *Lab. Invest.*, **31**, 516–532.

2. Kohaut, E. C., Singer, D. B., Nevels, B. K. and Hill, L. L. (1976). The specificity of split renal membranes in hereditary nephritis. *Arch. Pathol. Lab. Med.*, **100**, 475–479.

3. McCoy, R. C., Johnson, H. K., Stone, W. H. and Wilson, C. B. (1976). Variation in glomerular basement membrane antigens in hereditary nephritis (Abstract). *Lab. Invest.*, **34**, 325–326.

4. Gaboardi, F., Edefonti, A., Imbasciati, E., Tarantino, A., Mihatsch, M. J. and Zollinger, H. U. (1974). Alport's syndrome. Progressive hereditary nephritis. *Clin. Nephrol.*, **2**, 143–156.

5. Huttunen, N. P. (1976). Congenital nephrotic syndrome of Finnish type: Study of 75 patients. *Arch. Dis. Child.*, **51**, 344–348.

Index